Respiratory Medicine

Series editor

Sharon I.S. Rounds

More information about this series at http://www.springer.com/series/7665

Lynn M. Schnapp · Carol Feghali-Bostwick
Editors

Acute Lung Injury and Repair

Scientific Fundamentals and Methods

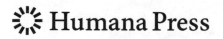 Humana Press

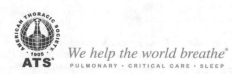

Editors
Lynn M. Schnapp, MD
Pulmonary, Critical Care, Allergy and Sleep
  Medicine
Medical University of South Carolina
Charleston, SC
USA

Carol Feghali-Bostwick, PhD
Division of Rheumatology and Immunology
Medical University of South Carolina
Charleston, SC
USA

ISSN 2197-7372   ISSN 2197-7380   (electronic)
Respiratory Medicine
ISBN 978-3-319-83535-8   ISBN 978-3-319-46527-2   (eBook)
DOI 10.1007/978-3-319-46527-2

Printed on acid-free paper

This Humana Press imprint is published by Springer Nature
The registered company is Springer International Publishing AG
The registered company address is: Gewerbestrasse 11, 6330 Cham, Switzerland

Contents

Contributors

William A. Altemeier, MD Division of Pulmonary and Critical Care Medicine, Department of Medicine, Center for Lung Biology, University of Washington, Seattle, WA, USA

Yu-Hua Chow, PhD Division of Pulmonary and Cricial Care Medicine, University of Washington School of Medicine, Seattle, WA, USA

Franco R. D'Alessio, MD Division of Pulmonary and Critical Care Medicine, Johns Hopkins Asthma and Allergy Center, Baltimore, MD, USA

Carol Feghali-Bostwick, PhD Division of Rheumatology, Medical University of South Carolina, Charleston, SC, USA

Lindsey M. Felton, BS Division of Pulmonary, Critical Care, Allergy, and Sleep Medicine, Medical University of South Carolina, Charleston, SC, USA

Andrew J. Goodwin, MD, MS Division of Pulmonary, Critical Care, Allergy and Sleep Medicine, Medical University of South Carolina, Charleston, SC, USA

Xiaozhu Huang, MD Department of Medicine, University of California, San Francisco, CA, USA

Chi F. Hung, MD Division of Pulmonary and Critical Care Medicine, Department of Medicine, Center for Lung Biology, University of Washington, Seattle, WA, USA

Melanie Königshoff, MD, PhD Comprehensive Pneumology Center (CPC), Helmholtz Zentrum Munich and Ludwig-Maximilians-University Munich, Munich, Germany

Emma Lefrançais, PhD Department of Medicine, University of California, San Francisco, San Francisco, CA, USA

Mark R. Looney, MD Department of Medicine, University of California, San Francisco, San Francisco, CA, USA

Beñat Mallavia, PhD Department of Medicine, University of California, San Francisco, San Francisco, CA, USA

Gustavo Matute-Bello, MD Division of Pulmonary and Critical Care Medicine, Department of Medicine, Center for Lung Biology, University of Washington, Seattle, WA, USA

Jason R. Mock, MD, PhD Division of Pulmonary Diseases and Critical Care Medicine, University of North Carolina School of Medicine, Chapel Hill, NC, USA

Kathrin Mutze, PhD Comprehensive Pneumology Center (CPC), Helmholtz Zentrum Munich and Ludwig-Maximilians-University Munich, Munich, Germany

Annette Robichaud, PhD SCIREQ Scientific Respiratory Equipment Inc., Montreal, QC, Canada

Lynn M. Schnapp, MD Division of Pulmonary, Crticial Care, Allergy and Sleep Medicine, Medical University of South Carolina, Charleston, SC, USA

Benjamin D. Singer, MD Division of Pulmonary and Critical Care Medicine, Northwestern University Feinberg School of Medicine, Chicago, IL, USA

Carole L. Wilson, PhD Division of Pulmonary, Critical Care, Allergy, and Sleep Medicine, Medical University of South Carolina, Charleston, SC, USA

Ivana V. Yang, PhD Department of Medicine, University of Colorado Anschutz Medical Campus, Aurora, USA; Department of Epidemiology, Colorado School of Public Health, Aurora, USA; Center for Genes, Environment, and Health, National Jewish Health, Denver, USA

Chapter 1
Methods to Study Lung Injury and Repair: Introduction

Lynn M. Schnapp and Carol Feghali-Bostwick

ARDS Overview

The acute respiratory distress syndrome (ARDS), first described in 1967 by Ashbaugh and colleagues [1], continues to have up to 40 % mortality, representing over 10 % of intensive care unit (ICU) admissions worldwide [2, 3]. Furthermore, the incidence is predicted to increase with the aging population [4]. Several clinical disorders can initiate ARDS, including pneumonia, sepsis, gastric aspiration, and trauma. The diagnostic criteria for ARDS have varied over time, which has led to different reports of incidence, morbidity, and mortality. The 2013 "Berlin Definition" was a consensus statement created by a task force of ARDS experts that built upon the 1994 AECC American-European Consensus Conference's definition statement [5]. The "Berlin Definition" of ARDS includes acute onset (<1 week), bilateral infiltrates on imaging, hypoxemia despite positive pressure ventilation and absence of congestive heart failure (Fig. 1.1). The clinical term "Acute Lung Injury (ALI)" has been replaced by mild, moderate or severe ARDS. This consensus definition has improved the standardization of clinical research and trials; however, it does not take into account the cause, or the mechanism of disease. Developing a molecular classification of the disease is needed to improve diagnosis, prognostication, and treatment.

L.M. Schnapp (✉)
Division of Pulmonary, Crtical Care, Allergy and Sleep Medicine,
Medical University of South Carolina, Charleston, SC, USA
e-mail: schnapp@musc.edu

C. Feghali-Bostwick
Division of Rheumatology, Medical University of South
Carolina, Charleston, SC, USA
e-mail: feghalib@musc.edu

© Springer International Publishing AG 2017
L.M. Schnapp and C. Feghali-Bostwick (eds.), *Acute Lung Injury and Repair*,
Respiratory Medicine, DOI 10.1007/978-3-319-46527-2_1

Fig. 1.1 Typical ARDS chest radiograph showing bilateral, patchy infiltrates. Courtesy of Dr. Andrew Goodwin, MUSC

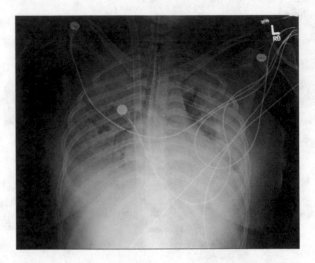

ARDS Pathogenesis

ARDS is characterized as an acute diffuse, inflammatory lung injury, leading to increased pulmonary vascular permeability, decreased lung compliance, and loss of aerated lung tissue leading to severe perturbations in gas exchange. The classic histological finding of ARDS is diffuse alveolar damage with edema, inflammation, and hyaline membrane formation [6]. During the early, exudative stage (days 1–7), the pathology is dominated by diffuse alveolar damage, epithelial injury and apoptosis, with significant inflammatory infiltration, and disruption of the capillary and epithelial barrier function with resultant interstitial and intraalveolar edema. In the later fibroproliferative stage, fibroblast proliferation, activation and migration dominate, with type II cell hyperplasia, and fibroproliferation. Interestingly, the majority of patients have resolution of fibroproliferation and pulmonary function improves over time. One of the unanswered questions in ARDS is what determines whether lung injury resolves or progresses to end-stage fibrosis? Why does fibroproliferation in ARDS resolve, but not in other chronic fibrosing diseases such as Idiopathic Pulmonary Fibrosis?

Therapeutic Options

The mainstay of treatment of ARDS remains supportive, including avoidance of iatrogenic injury. The ARDS Network trials demonstrated improved outcomes with low tidal volume mechanical ventilation [7], positive end-expiratory pressure [8], and conservative fluid management [9]. However, despite the presence of acute inflammation and role of inflammatory cells such as neutrophils [10], trials targeting the inflammatory process have failed to show definitive clinical benefit [2].

Specific therapeutics tested in clinical trials include corticosteroids, prostaglandins, nitric oxide, prostacyclin, surfactant, lisofylline, ketoconazole, N-acetylcysteine, granulocyte macrophage colony-stimulating factor, procysteine, indomethacin, simvastatin, pentoxyfilline, activated protein C and fish oil, none of which have shown a statistically significant improvement in mortality, despite promising pre-clinical trials in animal models [2]. Thus, new treatment options for ARDS remain a major unmet need.

Summary

Despite intense research over the past 40 years, we still have an incomplete understanding of the pathophysiology of the disease. Furthermore, treatment remains largely supportive. Future progress will depend on developing novel therapeutics that can facilitate and enhance lung repair. Because ARDS is a complex syndrome with a broad clinical phenotype, it has been challenging to translate the results of cell and animal studies to pharmacologic therapies that reduce mortality in humans [11, 12]. Nevertheless, laboratory-based investigations have produced valuable insights into the mechanisms responsible for the pathogenesis and resolution of lung injury, and preclinical studies paved the way for important improvements in supportive care. Currently, the use of mesenchymal stem cells for severe ARDS (NCT01775774) is being tested in a phase 2 clinical trial for ARDS, based on promising animal studies, and in vitro and ex vivo data [13]. Understanding the appropriate uses of animal models and in vitro studies, as well as defining the pathophysiologic subtypes of acute lung injury are necessary for the field to move forward from the descriptive phase of ARDS.

The chapters in this book describe various methodologies that are of particular utility in acute lung injury and repair research. They include descriptions of genetically engineered and non-engineered rodent models of ARDS. Although animal models of ARDS do not completely recapitulate all features of the human disease, these ALI models offer a means of testing potential therapies and possible initiating factors. Detailed protocols for establishing animal models and evaluation of lung injury are described (*chapters by Altemeier, Hung, Wilson, Huang, Konigshoff*). Flow cytometry approaches and their application to lung research are also detailed (*chapter by D'Alessio*). Novel approaches recently implemented in ALI research such as genomic approaches (*chapter by Yang*), the detection of miRNA (*chapter by Goodwin*), and imaging (*chapter by Looney*) are highlighted. Technical approaches such as flow cytometry are also presented in sufficient detail to facilitate adapting the protocols in laboratories less familiar with the methodology. We hope this book will serve as a very useful resource for physicians and scientists who are looking to develop strategies for insight into ARDS pathogenesis and treatment.

References

1. Ashbaugh DG, Bigelow DB, Petty TL, Levine BE. Acute respiratory distress in adults. Lancet. 1967;2:319–23.
2. Phua J, Badia JR, Adhikari NK, et al. Has mortality from acute respiratory distress syndrome decreased over time?: a systematic review. Am J Respir Crit Care Med. 2009;179:220–7.
3. Bellani G, Laffey JG, Pham T, et al. Epidemiology, patterns of care, and mortality for patients with acute respiratory distress syndrome in intensive care units in 50 countries. JAMA. 2016;315:788–800.
4. Rubenfeld GD, Caldwell E, Peabody E, et al. Incidence and outcomes of acute lung injury. N Engl J Med. 2005;353:1685–93.
5. The ADTF. Acute respiratory distress syndrome: the Berlin definition. JAMA. 2012;307:2526–33.
6. Matthay MA, Ware LB, Zimmerman GA. The acute respiratory distress syndrome. J Clin Invest. 2012;122:2731–40.
7. Network TARDS. Ventilation with lower tidal volumes as compared with traditional tidal volumes for acute lung injury and the acute respiratory distress syndrome. The Acute Respiratory Distress Syndrome Network. N Engl J Med 2000;342:1301–8.
8. Briel M, Meade M, Mercat A, et al. Higher vs lower positive end-expiratory pressure in patients with acute lung injury and acute respiratory distress syndrome: systematic review and meta-analysis. JAMA. 2010;303:865–73.
9. The National Heart L, Network BIARDSCT. Comparison of two fluid-management strategies in acute lung injury. N Engl J Med 2006;354:2564–75.
10. Bdeir K, Higazi AA, Kulikovskaya I, et al. Neutrophil alpha-defensins cause lung injury by disrupting the capillary-epithelial barrier. Am J Respir Crit Care Med. 2010;181:935–46.
11. Bastarache JA, Blackwell TS. Development of animal models for the acute respiratory distress syndrome. Dis Model Mech. 2009;2:218–23.
12. Matute-Bello G, Frevert CW, Martin TR. Animal models of acute lung injury. Am J Physiol Lung Cell Mol Physiol. 2008;295:L379–99.
13. Matthay MA, Goolaerts A, Howard JP, Lee JW. Mesenchymal stem cells for acute lung injury: preclinical evidence. Crit Care Med. 2010;38:S569–73.

Chapter 2
Mouse Models of Acute Lung Injury

William A. Altemeier, Chi F. Hung and Gustavo Matute-Bello

Introduction

Acute Respiratory Distress Syndrome or ARDS is a diffuse inflammatory lung process that frequently manifests in critically ill patients, with an estimated incidence of 190,000 cases and 74,500 deaths per year in the United States alone [1]. Clinical ARDS is associated with specific risk factors that can be broadly divided into intra-pulmonary conditions, including pneumonia, aspiration, and blunt trauma; and extra-pulmonary risk factors, including extra-pulmonary sepsis, trauma, significant blood product resuscitation, and pancreatitis [2]. Interestingly, ARDS frequently develops up to 72 h after hospital presentation and frequently in the setting of mechanical ventilation, suggesting that mechanical ventilation may play a role in the initiation of lung injury [3, 4]. Clinically, ARDS is manifested by bilateral or diffuse radiographic infiltrates, hypoxemia, decreased lung compliance, and increased ventilatory dead space [5, 6]. The histological manifestation of ARDS is diffuse alveolar damage as defined by epithelial injury, hyaline membrane formation and alveolar flooding with proteinaceous fluid, formation of microthrombi and frequently neutrophilic inflammation.

The animal model correlate to ARDS is acute lung injury (ALI). Models are employed to test potential new therapeutic interventions and to investigate underlying mechanistic pathways that lead to diffuse lung injury. Animal models cannot completely recapitulate all of the complex components of ARDS development and

W.A. Altemeier (✉) · C.F. Hung · G. Matute-Bello
Division of Pulmonary and Critical Care Medicine, Department of Medicine,
Center for Lung Biology, University of Washington, Seattle, WA, USA
e-mail: billa@uw.edu

C.F. Hung
e-mail: cfhung@uw.edu

G. Matute-Bello
e-mail: matuteb@uw.edu

© Springer International Publishing AG 2017
L.M. Schnapp and C. Feghali-Bostwick (eds.), *Acute Lung Injury and Repair*,
Respiratory Medicine, DOI 10.1007/978-3-319-46527-2_2

manifestation; however, an American Thoracic Society workshop concluded that animal models of ALI should at a minimum manifest histological evidence of tissue injury, alveolar capillary breakdown, inflammation, and physiological evidence of dysfunction with the first two components being more important than the last two [7]. The goals of this chapter are to discuss practical considerations when planning to utilize mouse models of acute lung injury and review some of the primary issues surrounding specific model systems.

Initial Considerations When Planning to Use Animal Models of Acute Lung Injury

Choice of Species/Strain/Sex

No animal model of acute lung injury can completely recapitulate clinical ARDS; therefore, when planning an experiment, the most important goal is determining which model system is most appropriate to address the underlying hypothesis being tested. The first consideration is choice of species. Mice have several well-defined advantages and disadvantages. The primary benefits of mice include the availability of genetic models to test specific mechanisms, the short reproductive cycle that allows rapid expansion of well-defined mouse populations, a large number of reagents available for mice, and lower cost as compared with other species. The primary disadvantages of mice include small size, which significantly increases the complexity of physiological monitoring and any surgical preparations, some immune system differences from humans, notably the lack of IL-8, and a general over-reliance on a limited number of inbred mouse strains when a specific genetic background is not required for testing the experimental hypothesis. Because the focus of this chapter is on mouse models of lung injury, the remainder of the discussion will be focused on mice; however, investigators are advised to consider larger animals, which allow more complete physiological monitoring and assessment, if the unique advantages of mice are not required for the planned study.

Genetic background is an important determinant of host response to both infectious lung injury [8, 9] and sterile lung injury [10–15]. Therefore, findings in a specific strain of inbred mouse, e.g., C57BL/6 or BALB/c, may not be applicable to other mouse strains much less other mammalian species. One common approach to overcome the potential confounding effect of limited genetic variation in experiments that do not require a specific genetic background (e.g., pharmacological or toxicological studies) is to employ outbred mouse stocks, e.g., Swiss outbred mice (stock refers to colonies of outbred mice; whereas, strains are used to define colonies of inbred mice). However, a criticism of this approach is that the genetic variability in these stocks can vary widely depending on the source and prior breeding strategies and are not well-defined [16]. Additionally, genetic lability in these populations may make it difficult to accurately estimate sample sizes based on previously published experimental results. Therefore, experiments using outbred stock typically require significantly larger sample sizes, which need to be empirically determined in preliminary studies. An alternative approach to using outbred stock is a factorial experimental design, which uses smaller sample sizes in multiple inbred lines, allowing evaluation of the impact of genetic variability on the measured variables [17].

Similar to genetic background, sex can have a significant impact on experimental response to injury and, presumably, to any interventions. For example, sex likely impacts response to prolonged hyperoxia. In our unpublished experience, female C57BL/6 mice are more susceptible to hyperoxia-induce lung injury than male mice. This is consistent with a recent publication, demonstrating a modest increase in mortality with prolonged hyperoxia in female C57BL/6 mice and female mice from the F1 cross of C57BL/6J mice (susceptible to hyperoxia) and 129X1/SvJ mice (resistant to hyperoxia) [18]. In contrast, other groups have found greater susceptibility to hyperoxia-induced lung injury in male mice [19, 20], suggesting that sex effects are complex and may interact with multiple other factors, including strain and environment. Another example of the effect of sex on lung injury models is the finding that C57BL/6 male mice are reported to be more susceptible to bleomycin-induced lung injury [21, 22], which is consistent with unpublished findings from our lab. However, female Fisher rats are reported to be more susceptible to bleomycin-induced fibrosis than male rats [23]. The etiology of sex-based differences in lung injury response is often attributed to sex hormones, and several studies have evaluated this but yielded limited mechanistic insight. Given these results, it is tempting to identify the more responsive sex for the particular model of interest and then use only this sex in the experimental design to reduce overall number of animals required. However, the NIH has recently emphasized the importance of including both sexes in preclinical studies unless a strong rationale can be provided for only studying one sex [24].

In summary, the primary advantages of using mice to model acute lung injury are the ability to utilize genetic systems to isolate and evaluate specific mechanistic hypotheses, the wide availability of reagents, and low cost. If a specific genetic strain is not required for the experiments, there may be advantages to evaluating a limited number of inbred mouse strains to both evaluate the potential impact of genetics on the response to injury and to decrease the likelihood that a specific genotype may be associated with hyporesponsiveness to any tested interventions. Similarly, both sexes should be included in experimental design unless a compelling reason exists to exclude one sex. However, data analysis should include evaluating the potential of a sex model interaction.

Choice of Lung Injury Model

ARDS is associated with a variety of pre-disposing conditions, which can be categorized as either direct injury (e.g., pneumonia, aspiration, pulmonary contusion) or indirect (sepsis, trauma, transfusion) or indirect injury. Accordingly, there are models that utilize direct injury (e.g., bacterial, viral, lipopolysaccharide (LPS), or acid instillation) and models that utilize indirect injury (e.g., cecal ligation and puncture (CLP), intraperitoneal LPS injection, transfusion associated lung injury). However, generally models utilizing an extra-pulmonary trigger for lung injury result in at most mild lung injury in the absence of a second insult such as mechanical ventilation. For example, CLP, a model of severe sepsis that is associated with significant mortality, results in minimal lung injury in mice [25]. In contrast, models of lung injury that rely on a direct pulmonary insult cause reproducible injury that can be readily titrated by exposure dose/duration. The addition of mechanical ventilation increases lung injury to most if not all direct models of lung injury, including instillation of LPS and other pathogen-associated molecular patterns (PAMP) [26–28], bacterial pneumonia [29], acid instillation [30, 31], and hyperoxia [32]. Because the majority of lung injury models utilize a direct exposure, the remainder of this chapter will review the more common model systems. The focus will be on practical issues necessary to initiate different model systems in a lab. Individuals interested in further reading regarding mechanisms of lung injury with different models are referred to a previously published review as a starting reference [33].

Instillation of Pathogen-Associated Molecular Patterns

Instillation of natural or synthetic pathogen-associated molecular patterns (PAMPs), which are recognized by specific germ-line encoded pattern recognition receptors (e.g., Toll-like receptors or TLRs) causes reproducible sterile lung inflammation and injury. The most common PAMP used is lipopolysaccharide (LPS), a component of the cell walls of gram-negative bacteria. LPS binds to its cognate receptor, TLR4 and the co-receptor, CD14. However, LPS is available in a variety of preparations, which may contain varying contamination with other pathogen-associated molecular patterns. Thus, ultra-pure LPS, available from select companies (e.g., Invivogen or List Biological Laboratories), will not cause inflammation in the absence of TLR4. In contrast, many sources of LPS will contain impurities that signal via additional TLRs. In our experience, the potency in terms of inflammation and injury is typically higher for lower purity preparations, presumably due to parallel signaling by multiple pattern recognition receptors. We routinely use phenol-extracted LPS from *Escherichia coli* 0111:B4, purchased from Sigma-Aldrich. We resuspend LPS at 5 mg/mL in sterile saline. Heating to 37 °C and/or sonication can facilitate resuspension of LPS. Aliquots of stock solution can then be stored at −20 °C indefinitely.

LPS is easily administered via oropharyngeal aspiration, and a detailed protocol is provided below. The dose of LPS can be titrated to achieve the desired degree of inflammation and injury. For phenol-extracted LPS from *E. coli* 0111:B4 purchased from Sigma-Aldrich, a dose of 2.5–3.75 mg/kg results in moderate lung injury that peaks in 48–72 h and resolves by 10 days (Fig. 2.1) [34, 35]. Other PAMPs, e.g., poly(I:C), a synthetic analog of dsRNA and TLR3 ligand, and Pam3CSK4 a

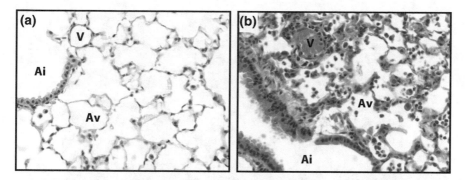

Fig. 2.1 Hematoxylin and Eosin stained, formalin-fixed lung sections from mice exposed by oropharyngeal aspiration 72 h previously to **a** phosphate-buffered saline or **b** 2.5 mg/kg of *E. coli* serotype 0111:B4 LPS. Note damage to the airway wall, thickening of alveolar septae, and inflammatory cell infilatrate, following LPS exposure. *Ai*—airway, *Av*—alveolus, *V*—vasculature. Note the alveolar septal thickening, alveolar inflammatory infiltrate, and airway wall injury in the LPS-exposed mouse lung

synthetic triacetylated lipoprotein and TLR1/2 ligand, can be administered by oropharyngeal aspiration to induce mild to moderate lung injury [28]. Similar to LPS, dose titration and a time course are recommended in preliminary experiments to define optimal experimental parameters.

Bacterial Pneumonia Models

Bacterial infection is a commonly used and clinically relevant model of lung injury. In addition to modeling neutrophilic inflammation and alveolar capillary barrier dysfunction, use of live bacteria allows assessment of additional relevant host response questions, including bacterial clearance and bacterial dissemination. These additional parameters are particularly important when assessing potential new therapeutic interventions, given that pneumonia and sepsis are two of the most common causes of ARDS. Mice have varying susceptibility to different bacteria. C57BL/6 mice will clear *Staphylococcus aureus* and *Pseudomonas aeruginosa* without antibiotics and will survive infections with relatively high bacterial loads of 10^6–10^7 [36]. In contrast mice are highly susceptible to *Klebsiella pneumonia*, and intratracheal inoculation of 700 cfu in CBA/J mice results in ~ 20 % mortality by 72 h [37].

Bacteria can be aerosolized and delivered via a whole body or nose-only exposure system or given by oropharyngeal aspiration. The advantages of aerosolization include dosing a large number of mice simultaneously and achieving a uniform deposition in the lung, however, the cost for setting up an aerosolization system can be significantly higher. We use the AeroMP aerosol management platform combined with a whole body exposure chamber (Biaera Technologies,

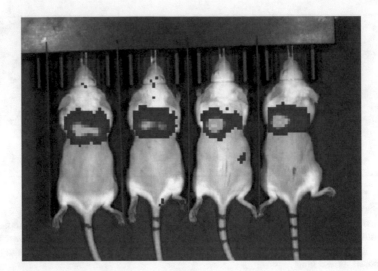

Fig. 2.2 Four mice imaged, using the IVIS in vivo imaging system 6 h after oropharyngeal administration of bioluminescent *P. aeruginosa* (Xen 05, Perkin Elmer). Mice are anesthetized with isoflurane and imaged in the supine posture. Note heterogeneous distribution typical of oropharyngeal aspiration in mouse 3 and mouse 4

Hagerstown, MD), but other systems, including non-commercial set-ups are also effective. Additionally, when delivering bacteria by aerosol, preliminary experiments, in which mice are euthanized immediately after exposure for quantitative cultures of the lungs are necessary to define the relationship between aerosolization parameters (concentration, duration) and deposition.

The primary advantage of oropharyngeal aspiration is the ability to quickly get an infection model up and running without the need to optimize delivery parameters to achieve the desired inoculation. Additionally, higher loads of bacteria can be delivered by direct inoculation as opposed to aerosolization (Fig. 2.2). Finally, an argument can be made that oropharyngeal aspiration, which results in heterogeneous infection, better models clinical pneumonia. An example protocol for preparing *S. aureus* for infection is provided at the end of this chapter.

Hyperoxia-Induced Lung Injury

Prolonged exposure to high oxygen fractions causes lung injury in a strain- and sex-dependent manner that is thought to be secondary to generation of reactive oxygen species, leading to peroxidation of membrane lipids, proteins, and nucleic acids and promotion of both necrotic and apoptotic cellular death [38]. In contrast to bacterial or LPS-induced lung injury, hyperoxia is associated primarily with disruption of the alveolar capillary barrier, and neutrophilic inflammation develops late in moribund mice. Exposure of female C57BL/6 mice to an inspired oxygen fraction of ≥ 0.95 results in measurable permeability changes by 36–48 h, neutrophilic emigration into the alveolar spaces by 72–84 h, and death by 96–120 h. In contrast, approximately 80 % of female C57BL/6 mice will survive exposure to an FiO_2 of ~ 0.8 [39]. Although hyperoxia exposure systems for mice are commercially available, it is also relatively straightforward to fashion one. A non-airtight Plexiglas box, sufficient to hold one or more micro-isolator mouse cages and with a hinged end for access, is connected to an oxygen concentrator, capable of delivering oxygen at 5 lpm. A vacuum line is also attached to the box with vacuum sufficient to result in ~ 3 lpm air flow. As long as the box is not airtight, oxygen delivery in excess of the flow through the vacuum system will vent to the room and also result in an elevated oxygen fraction in the chamber. However, in the event of failure of the oxygen concentrator, the vacuum line will pull sufficient fresh ambient air through the exposure chamber to prevent build-up of CO_2. Fine tuning of the actual oxygen concentration in the chamber can be achieved by adjusting the inspiratory oxygen flow and/or the vacuum flow.

Bleomycin-Induced Lung Injury

Bleomycin is an anti-neoplastic drug isolated from *Streptomyces verticillus* [40]. Intratracheal administration of bleomycin is typically thought of as a model of pulmonary fibrosis; however, in fact it causes injury that follows a well-defined pattern of acute neutrophilic inflammation and disruption of the alveolar capillary barrier that peaks by day 3–7 followed by resolution of inflammation and development of a fibroproliferative phase that peaks around day 21–24, which then resolves over time [41–43]. Dosing of bleomycin can be challenging; there is a narrow dose range in which significant lung injury develops, but the majority of animals recover. This is further complicated by a significant sex-dependent variation in susceptibility with female C57BL/6 mice being significantly more resistant to bleomycin-induced lung injury than male mice. A prudent practice is to prepare bleomycin in quantities sufficient to complete a series of experiments, aliquot and store at −20 °C, and then perform an initial dose response experiment to determine the optimal dose for that particular preparation. Additionally, because of the potential concern for injury to the pharynx and larynx, most investigators will intubate mice and administer bleomycin intratracheally as opposed to administration by oropharyngeal aspiration. Several different approaches to orally intubating mice have been described [44–46].

Ventilator-Induced Lung Injury

Mechanical ventilation is commonly employed, clinically, to support patients with ARDS. However, beginning in the 1990s, clinicians recognized that mechanical ventilation can also worsen injury in patients with ARDS, culminating in a large, multi-center trial that demonstrated a large mortality benefit associated with reducing tidal volumes in patients with ARDS [47]. Additionally, retrospective studies have suggested that mechanical ventilation can increase the likelihood of ARDS developing in patients with ARDS risk factors [3, 4]. Similarly, mechanical ventilation in mice will induce lung injury as measured by histological changes, neutrophilic inflammation, and disruption of the alveolar capillary barrier. Mouse models of mechanical ventilation have used large tidal volumes and low or absent positive end-expiratory pressure (PEEP) in isolation to induce lung injury; however, this approach is limited by several factors, including relative resistance of mice to lung injury from ventilation alone, potential impact on hemodynamics, which are challenging to quantify and adjust in mice, and questions regarding the clinical relevance of such models. In contrast, mechanical ventilation with moderate tidal volumes in the range of 10–15 mL/kg synergistically increases lung injury when combined with bacterial products [26, 28, 48], infections [29], hyperoxia [32], and acid instillation [30]. The mechanisms by which mechanical ventilation interacts with other forms of lung injury to amplify the injury response are unclear and remains an active area of investigation. Mechanical ventilation, using parameters that do not result in overt lung injury, results in transcriptional activation of pathways associated with inflammation and may synergistically upregulate pro-inflammatory mediators associated with lung injury and development of extra-pulmonary organ dysfunction [29, 49–52]. Additionally, mechanical strain likely causes physical disruption of cellular membranes, particularly in lung epithelial cells [53, 54], resulting in release of damage-associated molecular patterns and inflammatory activation [28]. Mechanical ventilation in mice is technically challenging, particularly for periods longer than 4 h. A number of pitfalls can significantly increase mortality. For example, body temperature is difficult to regulate in a mouse that is anesthetized and supine, and typical warming pads placed under the mice are insufficient. Temperature regulation is better if the mouse is prone on a warming pad but limits access to the mouse. We have found that a heat lamp with a rheostat is the most effective method for maintaining body temperature of mechanically ventilated mice in the supine posture. However, body temperature must be monitored via a rectal thermistor or similar method to insure that it remains within an appropriate range. A second important issue is control of mouse respiratory effort. In our experience, total suppression of mouse respiratory effort is not feasible with anesthesia alone. Given that mouse ventilators generally are simple volume adjustable syringe pistons with a user set frequency, discordance between spontaneous respiratory effort and the ventilator's respiratory cycle are inevitable. This is easily observed as variation in airway pressure over short intervals. To prevent spontaneous respiratory effort, neuromuscular paralysis with a non-depolarizing paralytic agent, such as pancuronium, vecuronium, or rocuronium is required. Such agents require a plan for monitoring adequacy of anesthesia, which is challenging in a paralyzed mouse. Our experience is that non-invasive blood pressure measurements are unreliable in anesthetized, mechanically ventilated mice. Invasive monitoring of blood pressure would be sufficient but is technically challenging and significantly increases preparation time and risk of unintended death. One option is to monitor heart rate via EKG and develop an algorithm with the Institutional Animal Care and Use Committee to identify parameters for anesthesia adjustment. For example, increases in heart rate of 20 % or more could trigger an increase in inhaled isoflurane concentration by 0.5 % or an additional dose of systemic anesthetic at half the original induction dose. Finally, monitoring for continued mouse viability is important. In our experience, anesthetized, paralyzed, ventilated mice can die on the ventilator without recognition by performing personnel. If airway pressure is monitored, then a rapid, large increase in airway pressure typically signals death. However, measurements that are more robust include monitoring exhaled CO_2 or monitoring the EKG. A general description of a mouse mechanical ventilation setup is included at the end of this chapter.

Assessment of Lung Injury

A comprehensive workshop report by the American Thoracic Society has been published outlining assessment of lung injury in animal models and should be referred to for an in-depth discussion [7]. However, to summarize, the primary features of experimental acute lung injury in animals were identified as histological evidence of tissue injury, alteration of the alveolar capillary barrier, evidence of an inflammatory response, and evidence of physiological dysfunction. Of these parameters, quantitative assessment of alveolar capillary barrier and quantitative assessment of inflammation are the most commonly employed and easiest to measure. In our opinion, histological evidence of lung injury is most useful for a qualitative demonstration of injury and to identify potential anatomical localizations of specific processes, e.g., by IHC. This position paper proposed a semi-quantitative histology system that has been commonly employed; however, without a systematic sampling system such as designed-based stereology, the quantitative value of this approach is questionable [55].

Multiple approaches can be used to assess alveolar capillary barrier integrity, including assessment of extravascular fluid accumulation and permeability of the lung to macromolecules. The most common measure of extravascular fluid accumulation is wet lung weight at the time of necropsy, normalized either to the dry lung weight, obtained by drying the lung in an oven until weight no longer changes, or to pre-experiment total body weight. Disruption of the alveolar capillary barrier is commonly measured by presence of serum proteins in the alveolar compartment. The simplest, yet reliable, measure is to assay total protein in cell-free bronchoalveolar lavage fluid by the bicinchoninic acid or BCA assay. A brief protocol for mouse bronchoalveolar lavage is included at the end of this chapter. Another approach is to quantify IgM in bronchoalveolar lavage fluid, using a commercially available ELISA (e.g., Bethyl Laboratories). IgM exists in a pentameric form with a molecular weight of ~ 900 kD. It is not normally present in the alveolar compartment, and elevated levels imply frank disruption of the alveolar capillary barrier. Other techniques include injecting mice with Evan's Blue dye at a dose of 20 mg/kg. Evan's Blue dye labels albumin, in vivo, and translocates to the lung with albumin during lung injury. Permeability is then measured by flushing the pulmonary vasculature via the right ventricle, post-mortem, extracting the dye with formamide, quantifying by spectrophotometry [56]. An additional method is to intravenously inject mice with 100 μL of a 14.4 mM solution of a fluorescence-labeled 70 kD dextran (ThermoFisher Scientific) 1–3 h prior to euthanasia. Injections are most consistently accomplished via the retro orbital sinus in anesthetized mice. Degree of alveolar capillary permeability can be assessed by measuring the specific fluorescent label in bronchoalveolar fluid with a fluorimeter [28].

Assessment of cellular lung inflammation is easily assessed in bronchoalveolar lavage fluid. Because the number of cells present in the alveolar compartment of normal lungs are relatively low, counting can be facilitated by spinning out the cells from the lavage fluid and then suspending them in a smaller volume (0.2–0.5 mL). Total cell count is made using a hemocytometer, and percentage of neutrophils and mononuclear cells can be assessed on a cytospin preparation of 30,000 cells, using a modified Wright stain. Percentages of other cell types, such as lymphocytes and eosinophils are also often made; however, reliably distinguishing these specific cell types can be challenging and flow cytometry analysis should be considered. Release of pro-inflammatory cytokines can also be assessed via standard ELISA or multiplex assays on cell-free bronchoalveolar lavage fluid as well as tissue homogenate.

Assessment of physiological dysfunction is the most challenging lung injury parameter to obtain in mice. Measurement of gas exchange can be attempted with trans-cutaneous oximeters; however, these devices are frequently unreliable in anesthetized mice. We have found that the best reading is obtained on a mouse thigh after removing hair by a depilatory. Arterial blood gas measurements can also be attempted via left ventricular cardiac puncture. More recently, computer-controlled mechanical ventilators have been developed (e.g., flexiVent, SciReq), which allow application of defined forced oscillatory waveforms to mice. Measurement of pressure fluctuations with changing volume allows estimation of lung mechanics, including elastance and resistance [57]. These newer ventilators also allow measurement of more traditional pressure–volume curves for estimating lung compliance.

Many of these measures can be done in the same animal and a general guideline is that measuring lung injury by multiple different methods will increase confidence in the overall conclusions of the study. We routinely combine measurements of elastance over time, lung extravascular water as estimated by lung weight normalized to body weight, alveolar capillary disruption by measurement of total protein, IgM concentration, and extravasation of 70 kD fluorescence-labeled dextran, leukocyte total and subset counts in the bronchoalveolar lavage fluid, and assessment of pro-inflammatory cytokine release in bronchoalveolar lavage fluid.

Example Protocols

Oropharyngeal Aspiration (Fig. 2.3)

Materials needed

- Stand for suspending a mouse via front incisors (available commercially but a metal bookend, bent to a 75° angle with a rubber band stretched between two bolts works well)
- Two small forceps
- 200 µL pipet
- Anesthesia.

Oropharyngeal aspiration is a straightforward and relatively quick method to deliver material to the lungs. The primary limitation to this method is that distribution of material to the lungs is heterogeneous with a tendency toward greater delivery to the left lung. In a study comparing oropharyngeal aspiration to intratracheal instillation and nose-only aerosol delivery, the fractional distribution of a [99m]technetium-labled sulfur colloid to the lungs by oropharyngeal aspiration was equivalent to that of intratracheal instillation and significantly higher than that observed with aerosolization [58]. Importantly, the optimal volume for aspiration in this study was identified as ~ 50 µL.

For oropharyngeal instillation, prepare the instillate at a concentration for which 50 µL or 2 µL/g body weight of the mouse will result in the desired dose. Load 50 µL or 2 µL/g body weight into a P200 pipet. Anesthetize the mouse. Although systemic anesthesia such as ketamine/xylazine will work, use of an inhaled anesthetic such as isoflurane in an exposure chamber provides adequate duration of anesthesia for the procedure and results in more rapid recovery of the mouse. The level of anesthesia should be sufficient that the mouse is unresponsive to handling,

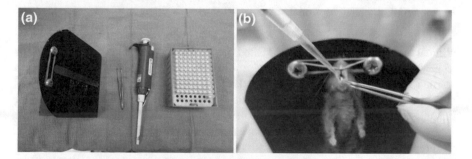

Fig. 2.3 Setup for oropharyngeal aspiration. **a** Equipment needed from *left* to *right* include an angled stand from which to suspend a mouse by its front incisors, a curved micro-forceps, a 200 µl pipet with aersol-resistant tips. **b** Anesthetized mice are suspended by their front incisors. The tongue is gently extended with the forceps, and 50 µl of instillate is introduced to the oropharynx. The tongue must be kept extended until the liquid is completely aspirated (~ 20 respiratory cycles)

and respiratory rate has decreased and is notably deeper. At this level of anesthesia, the mouse is suspended by its front incisors from the stand. Using the two forceps, the oral cavity is exposed and the tongue is fully extended. This is a critical step as lack of tongue extension will result in swallowing of the instilled material as opposed to aspiration. The pressure exerted with the forceps must be sufficient to keep the tongue fully extended without causing significant tissue trauma, resulting in edema and impairment of subsequent food and water intake. Once the tongue is extended, the pipet tip is inserted into the posterior oropharynx and the liquid is instilled. At this point, the tongue must be kept extended until the liquid is fully aspirated as determined visually by clearance from the oropharyngeal cavity. Our practice is to typically keep the tongue extended for 5 breaths following clearance of the liquid from the oropharynx. Failure to keep the tongue extended during this period will result in variable amounts of the instillate being ingested as opposed to aspirated. Following instillation, the mouse is removed and recovered from anesthesia.

Protocol for Preparing S. aureus

Materials needed

- *S. aureus* stock (commercial or clinical)
- Tryptic soy (TS) broth
- Sheep blood agar plates
- Sterile 50 % glycerol
- 100 mm Petri dishes
- 50 mL conical tubes
- sterile 250 mL Erlenmeyer flasks
- sterile 0.9 % saline
- sterile, distilled water
- spectrophotometer (optional).

To infect mice with *S. aureus*, first obtain bacteria from either a commercial or clinical source. Bacteria are then streaked out on a sheep blood agar plate and allow to grow until discrete colonies are present. Then, pick one colony with a loop or a sterile toothpick and inoculate into 50 mL of TS broth. Culture overnight in a 37 °C shaking incubator. The following morning, prepare *S. aureus* aliquots by adding 0.5 mL of bacterial suspension to 0.5 mL of sterile 40 % glycerol in a sterile screw-top tube and vortex. Glycerol stocks can then be stored at −80 °C for years. To prepare bacteria for experiments, thaw one aliquot and add 100 μl of *S. aureus* stock into 10 mL of TS broth. Incubate for 6 h in a 37 °C shaking incubator. Take 500 μL of this culture and add to 50 mL of TS broth and incubate for 16 h in a 37 °C shaking incubator.

To prepare the expanded culture for infection in mice, divide into two 50 mL conical tubes and add 25 mL of sterile 0.9 % saline to each tube, mixing thoroughly. Centrifuge at 3000 rpm for 15 min and remove supernatant. Re-suspend pellet in each tube with 1 mL of sterile saline and mix thoroughly. Add sterile saline up to 50 mL in each tube, and centrifuge at 3000 rpm for 15 min. Re-suspend each pellet again in 1 mL of saline and combine. Bring up to 50 mL with saline. Centrifuge at 3000 rpm for 15 min. Remove supernatant and re-suspend in 1 mL of sterile water. This should result in a stock of $\sim 10^{11}$ cfu/mL of *S. aureus* that is depleted of bacterial debris. However, to improve accuracy and consistency of bacterial dosing across experiments, a reasonable initial step is to prepare serial log dilutions of prepared stock in water. The turbidity is quickly measured by the OD_{540} for each dilution (be careful not to let the bacteria settle, which will affect the reading), and 100 μL of each dilution is added to bacterial culture plates with LB agar. Allow cultures to grow and count colonies. A standard curve can be prepared so that, with future experiments, the OD_{540} can be used to give consistent bacterial doses to mice.

Protocol for Mouse Mechanical Ventilation

Materials needed

- Mouse mechanical ventilator capable of delivering desired tidal volumes (e.g., 300 μL provides 12 ml/kg for a 25-g mouse). Typically, the syringe piston has a volume of 1 mL. A number of models are commercially available, ranging from simple volume cycled pistons with manually adjusted volumes and frequencies (e.g., mouse ventilator, Ugo Basile) to computer-controlled models that can apply various ventilator pertubations, allowing calculation of lung mechanics (e.g., flexiVent, SciReq).
- Positive end-expiratory pressure (PEEP) water column—can be as simple as a 50 mL conical tube with cap and an inlet through which expiratory tubing is passed into the water to the desired depth and an outlet (connected to a scavenging device if inhaled anesthetic used)
- Rectal thermistor probe for monitoring body temperature
- Electrodes and amplifier for monitoring EKG (may be included with computer-controlled ventilator systems or purchased separately (e.g., PowerLab system with Bio Amp, ADInstruments)
- Pressure transducer and amplifier for measuring pressure (may be included with computer-controlled ventilators or purchased separately (e.g., Bridge Amplifier, ADInstruments)
- Small animal isoflurane vaporizer (e.g., tabletop non-rebreathing anesthesia machine, Harvard Apparatus) with appropriate scavenging system (F/AIR canister or exhausted to fume hood)
- Anesthesia induction chamber

- Anesthesia nose cone delivery system
- Isoflurane
- Vecuronium
- Heating lamp with rheostat
- Endotracheal tube—(e.g., 0.5″ 18–20-gauge blunt needle with Luer stub adapter, VWR)
- Y connector and tubing to connect ventilator to endotracheal tube and endotracheal tube to PEEP chamber
- Microtip forceps ×2
- Microtip surgical scissors
- 4-0 silk suture.

Prior to intubation, mice are weighed to allow calculation of tidal volumes and drug doses. Mechanical ventilators should be set up prior to mouse anesthesia induction with appropriate ventilation parameters. In our system, we have found that a tidal volume of 12 mL/kg and a respiratory rate of 150 yields a left ventricular PCO_2 of approximately 35–45 mmHg. However, this is dependent on the dead space of the ventilator circuit and maintenance of a core body temperature between 36 and 38 °C. Additionally, changing the tidal volume will obviously require adjusting the rate. For any planned mechanical ventilation experiments, preliminary studies with arterial blood gas determination from left ventricular puncture is recommended to insure that appropriate ventilation is achieved. Determination of desired PEEP and adjustment of depth of exhaled gas tubing in the PEEP water column should also be done at this time. A typical value for mice that limits progressive atelectasis is a PEEP of 3 cm H_2O, requiring the tip of the exhaled gas tubing to be inserted 3 cm into the water column.

For anesthesia induction and intubation, our lab typically exposes a mouse to 5 % isoflurane for $\sim$3–4 min or until it is immobile with visually apparent reduced respiratory rate. The mouse is then removed to a nose cone exposure system, and anesthesia is maintained at 3 % isoflurane. Mouse limbs are secured with tape to a board, allowing full exposure of the ventral mouse. A midline skin incision is made over the neck and the trachea is bluntly dissected free with forceps. 4-0 silk suture is passed underneath the trachea. A T-shaped incision is made in the trachea, and the endotracheal tube is inserted and secured by tying the suture around the trachea, containing the endotracheal tube. The mouse is then quickly transferred to the mechanical ventilator, and ventilation is initiated with inhaled isoflurane at 1.5 %. Once in place, neuromuscular blockade is induced with vecuronium, 0.6 mg/kg, via intraperitoneal injection. This process requires either multiple isoflurane vaporizers or some planning and practice to switch the isoflurane flow from exposure chamber to nose cone delivery system, to mechanical ventilator inlet port. An alternative to this is to use a systemic anesthesia such as ketamine and xylazine for induction and then transition to isoflurane to maintain anesthesia during mechanical ventilation.

Once the mouse is secured on the ventilator, monitoring probes should be placed, including rectal thermistor probe and EKG leads. The initial body temperature will likely be less than 36 °C because of anesthesia induction and supine positioning during intubation. Re-warming with a heat lamp should be initiated as soon as possible and monitored closely to prevent over-warming. Initial heart rate with isoflurane anesthesia will be in the 350–500 range. If ketamine and xylazine are used, it will be in the 200–300 range due to negative chronotropic effects of xylazine. Airway pressures are typically in the 12–16 cm H_2O range. If they are significantly higher, this likely represents placement of the endotracheal tube tip against the airway wall, and careful repositioning of the mice may alleviate this issue.

For prolonged mechanical ventilation, airway pressures, heart rate, and body temperature should be monitored and recorded at a minimum of every 15 min. Continuous monitoring with audible alarms at set thresholds is safer. Body temperature should be maintained between 36 and 38 °C. Increases in heart rate of 20 % or higher prompt an increase in isoflurane by 0.5 % or re-dosing of systemic anesthesia at half the induction dose. Vecuronium or other neuromuscular blocking agent should be redosed at 50 % of the original dose if ventilator dysnchrony is observed—either visually by watching the mouse's chest movement or by observing breath to breath variation in peak and/or end-expiratory airway pressures. For prolonged ventilation beyond 4 h, consideration of i.p. fluids, e.g., 0.2 mL of sterile saline, can be considered to prevent hypovolemia and impaired perfusion. For mechanical ventilation beyond 4 h, particularly with volume resuscitation, we have noted the development of significantly reduced heart rate which can progress to cardiac arrest. This appears to be associated with urinary retention and bladder distension. If this is observed, the bladder can sometimes be palpated and expressed, resulting in normalization of the heart rate. At the conclusion of the planned ventilation period, mice are euthanized by anesthesia overdose followed by confirmatory sternotomy.

Post-mortem Bronchoalveolar Lavage Protocol

Materials needed

- 0.5″ 20-gauge blunt needle with Luer stub adapter (VWR)
- Microtip forceps ×2
- Microtip surgical scissors
- 4-0 silk suture
- 1 mL syringe
- Lavage fluid (e.g., PBS with 0.6 mM EDTA) warmed to 37 °C
- Eppendorf tubes
- Centrifuge.

After euthanasia, if the mouse is not already intubated, perform a midline incision in the skin over the neck. Using the forceps, bluntly dissect free the trachea and pass a piece of suture around it. Make a T incision, insert the 20-gauge blunt needle, and secure in place with the suture. To lavage both right and left lungs, gently instill 1 mL of lavage fluid, leave in place for 10 s, and then slowly withdraw until any resistance is met. Quantify the amount returned lavage fluid in the syringe and place in a collecting tube on ice. Bronchoalveolar lavage may then be repeated with pooling of returned fluid. Additional lavages increase the total number of cells collected but decreases the concentration of any proteins which may be of interest such as cytokines or IgM. A common practice is to perform lavage two or three times. However, if the goal is to obtain alveolar cells for subsequent analysis, then repeating lavage up to 5 times will increase yield.

Once all lavage samples are collected, place samples in a centrifuge at 4 °C and spin at $400 \times g$ for 5 min to pellet cells. The cell-free supernatant can then be removed, aliquoted, and stored at -80 °C for future assays. The cells are then suspended in 0.5 mL of PBS for counting and differential.

References

1. Rubenfeld GD, Caldwell E, Peabody E, Weaver J, Martin DP, Neff M, et al. Incidence and outcomes of acute lung injury. N Engl J Med. 2005;353:1685–93. doi:10.1056/NEJMoa050333.
2. Hudson LD, Milberg JA, Anardi D, Maunder RJ. Clinical risks for development of the acute respiratory distress syndrome. Am J Respir Crit Care Med. 1995;151:293–301.
3. Jia X, Malhotra A, Saeed M, Mark RG, Talmor D. Risk factors for ARDS in patients receiving mechanical ventilation for > 48 h. Chest. 2008;133:853–61. doi:10.1378/chest.07-1121.
4. Gajic O, Dara SI, Mendez JL, Adesanya AO, Festic E, Caples SM, et al. Ventilator-associated lung injury in patients without acute lung injury at the onset of mechanical ventilation. Crit Care Med. 2004;32:1817–24. doi:10.1097/01.CCM.0000133019.52531.30.
5. Ware LB, Matthay MA. The acute respiratory distress syndrome. N Engl J Med. 2000;342:1334–49. doi:10.1056/NEJM200005043421806.
6. ARDS Definition Task Force, Ranieri VM, Rubenfeld GD, Thompson BT, Ferguson ND, Caldwell E, et al. Acute respiratory distress syndrome: the Berlin Definition. 2012. p. 2526–33. doi:10.1001/jama.2012.5669.
7. Matute-Bello G, Downey G, Moore BB, Groshong SD, Matthay MA, Slutsky AS, et al. An official American Thoracic Society workshop report: features and measurements of experimental acute lung injury in animals. 2011. p. 725–38. doi:10.1165/rcmb.2009-0210ST.
8. Lorè NI, Iraqi FA, Bragonzi A. Host genetic diversity influences the severity of *Pseudomonas aeruginosa* pneumonia in the Collaborative Cross mice. BMC Genet. 2015;16:106. doi:10.1186/s12863-015-0260-6.
9. Ferris MT, Aylor DL, Bottomly D, Whitmore AC, Aicher LD, Bell TA, et al. Modeling host genetic regulation of influenza pathogenesis in the collaborative cross. PLoS Pathog. 2013;9: e1003196. doi:10.1371/journal.ppat.1003196.
10. Prows DR, Gibbons WJ, Smith JJ, Pilipenko V, Martin LJ. Age and sex of mice markedly affect survival times associated with hyperoxic acute lung injury. PLoS ONE. 2015;10: e0130936. doi:10.1371/journal.pone.0130936.
11. Rutledge H, Aylor DL, Carpenter DE, Peck BC, Chines P, Ostrowski LE, et al. Genetic regulation of Zfp30, CXCL1, and neutrophilic inflammation in murine lung. Genetics. 2014;198:735–45. doi:10.1534/genetics.114.168138.

12. Nichols JL, Gladwell W, Verhein KC, Cho H-Y, Wess J, Suzuki O, et al. Genome-wide association mapping of acute lung injury in neonatal inbred mice. FASEB J. 2014;28:2538–50. doi:10.1096/fj.13-247221.

13. Howden R, Cho H-Y, Miller-DeGraff L, Walker C, Clark JA, Myers PH, et al. Cardiac physiologic and genetic predictors of hyperoxia-induced acute lung injury in mice. Am J Respir Cell Mol Biol. 2012;46:470–8. doi:10.1165/rcmb.2011-0204OC.

14. Alm A-S, Li K, Chen H, Wang D, Andersson R, Wang X. Variation of lipopolysaccharide-induced acute lung injury in eight strains of mice. Respir Physiol Neurobiol. 2010;171:157–64. doi:10.1016/j.resp.2010.02.009.

15. Hudak BB, Zhang LY, Kleeberger SR. Inter-strain variation in susceptibility to hyperoxic injury of murine airways. Pharmacogenetics. 1993;3:135–43.

16. Chia R, Achilli F, Festing MFW, Fisher EMC. The origins and uses of mouse outbred stocks. Nat Genet. 2005;37:1181–6. doi:10.1038/ng1665.

17. Festing MFW. Principles: the need for better experimental design. Trends Pharmacol Sci. 2003;24:341–5. doi:10.1016/S0165-6147(03)00159-7.

18. Prows DR, Winterberg AV, Gibbons WJ, Burzynski BB, Liu C, Nick TG. Reciprocal backcross mice confirm major loci linked to hyperoxic acute lung injury survival time. Physiol Genomics. 2009;38:158–68. doi:10.1152/physiolgenomics.90392.2008.

19. Šarić A, Sobočanec S, Šafranko ŽM, Popović-Hadžija M, Aralica G, Korolija M, et al. Female headstart in resistance to hyperoxia-induced oxidative stress in mice. Acta Biochim Pol. 2014;61:801–7.

20. Lingappan K, Jiang W, Wang L, Couroucli XI, Moorthy B. Sex-specific differences in hyperoxic lung injury in mice: role of cytochrome P450 (CYP)1A. Toxicology. 2015;331:14–23. doi:10.1016/j.tox.2015.01.019.

21. Redente EF, Jacobsen KM, Solomon JJ, Lara AR, Faubel S, Keith RC, et al. Age and sex dimorphisms contribute to the severity of bleomycin-induced lung injury and fibrosis. Am J Physiol Lung Cell Mol Physiol. 2011;301:L510–8. doi:10.1152/ajplung.00122.2011.

22. Babin AL, Cannet C, Gérard C, Saint-Mezard P, Page CP, Sparrer H, et al. Bleomycin-induced lung injury in mice investigated by MRI: model assessment for target analysis. Magn Reson Med. 2012;67:499–509. doi:10.1002/mrm.23009.

23. Gharaee-Kermani M, Hatano K, Nozaki Y, Phan SH. Gender-based differences in bleomycin-induced pulmonary fibrosis. Am J Pathol. 2005;166:1593–606. doi:10.1016/S0002-9440(10)62470-4.

24. Clayton JA, Collins FS. Policy: NIH to balance sex in cell and animal studies. Nature. 2014;509:282–3.

25. Iskander KN, Craciun FL, Stepien DM, Duffy ER, Kim J, Moitra R, et al. Cecal ligation and puncture-induced murine sepsis does not cause lung injury. Crit Care Med. 2013;41:154–65. doi:10.1097/CCM.0b013e3182676322.

26. Altemeier WA, Matute-Bello G, Gharib SA, Glenny RW, Martin TR, Liles WC. Modulation of lipopolysaccharide-induced gene transcription and promotion of lung injury by mechanical ventilation. J Immunol. 2005;175:3369–76.

27. Hu G, Malik AB, Minshall RD. Toll-like receptor 4 mediates neutrophil sequestration and lung injury induced by endotoxin and hyperinflation. Crit Care Med. 2010;38:194–201. doi:10.1097/CCM.0b013e3181bc7c17.

28. Chun CD, Liles WC, Frevert CW, Glenny RW, Altemeier WA. Mechanical ventilation modulates Toll-like receptor-3-induced lung inflammation via a MyD88-dependent, TLR4-independent pathway: a controlled animal study. BMC Pulm Med. 2010;10:57. doi:10.1186/1471-2466-10-57.

29. Dhanireddy S, Altemeier WA, Matute-Bello G, O'Mahony DS, Glenny RW, Martin TR, et al. Mechanical ventilation induces inflammation, lung injury, and extra-pulmonary organ dysfunction in experimental pneumonia. Lab Invest. 2006;86:790–9. doi:10.1038/labinvest.3700440.

30. Gurkan OU, O'Donnell C, Brower R, Ruckdeschel E, Becker PM. Differential effects of mechanical ventilatory strategy on lung injury and systemic organ inflammation in mice. Am J Physiol Lung Cell Mol Physiol. 2003;285:L710–8. doi:10.1152/ajplung.00044.2003.

31. Allen GB, Leclair T, Cloutier M, Thompson-Figueroa J, Bates JHT. The response to recruitment worsens with progression of lung injury and fibrin accumulation in a mouse model of acid aspiration. Am J Physiol Lung Cell Mol Physiol. 2007;292:L1580–9. doi:10.1152/ajplung.00483.2006.

32. Makena PS, Luellen CL, Balazs L, Ghosh MC, Parthasarathi K, Waters CM, et al. Preexposure to hyperoxia causes increased lung injury and epithelial apoptosis in mice ventilated with high tidal volumes. Am J Physiol Lung Cell Mol Physiol. 2010;299:L711–9. doi:10.1152/ajplung.00072.2010.

33. Matute-Bello G, Frevert CW, Martin TR. Animal models of acute lung injury. Am J Physiol Lung Cell Mol Physiol. 2008;295:L379–99. doi:10.1152/ajplung.00010.2008.

34. D'Alessio FR, Tsushima K, Aggarwal NR, West EE, Willett MH, Britos MF, et al. CD4 +CD25+Foxp3+ Tregs resolve experimental lung injury in mice and are present in humans with acute lung injury. J Clin Invest. 2009;119:2898–913. doi:10.1172/JCI36498.

35. Klaff LS, Gill SE, Wisse BE, Mittelsteadt K, Matute-Bello G, Chen P, et al. Lipopolysaccharide-induced lung injury is independent of serum vitamin d concentration. PLoS ONE. 2012;7:e49076. doi:10.1371/journal.pone.0049076.

36. Skerrett SJ, Liggitt HD, Hajjar AM, Wilson CB. Cutting edge: myeloid differentiation factor 88 is essential for pulmonary host defense against *Pseudomonas aeruginosa* but not *Staphylococcus aureus*. J Immunol. 2004;172:3377–81.

37. Tsai WC, Strieter RM, Zisman DA, Wilkowski JM, Bucknell KA, Chen GH, et al. Nitric oxide is required for effective innate immunity against *Klebsiella pneumoniae*. Infect Immun. 1997;65:1870–5.

38. Altemeier WA, Sinclair SE. Hyperoxia in the intensive care unit: why more is not always better. Current Opin Crit Care. 2007;13:73–8. doi:10.1097/MCC.0b013e32801162cb.

39. Lozon TI, Eastman AJ, Matute-Bello G, Chen P, Hallstrand TS, Altemeier WA. PKR-dependent CHOP induction limits hyperoxia-induced lung injury. Am J Physiol Lung Cell Mol Physiol. 2011;300:L422–9. doi:10.1152/ajplung.00166.2010.

40. Umezawa H. Bleomycin and other antitumor antibiotics of high molecular weight. Antimicrob Agents Chemother. 1965;5:1079–85.

41. Gasse P, Mary C, Guenon I, Noulin N, Charron S, Schnyder-Candrian S, et al. IL-1R1/MyD88 signaling and the inflammasome are essential in pulmonary inflammation and fibrosis in mice. J Clin Invest. 2007;117:3786–99. doi:10.1172/JCI32285.

42. Xu J, Mora A, Shim H, Stecenko A, Brigham KL, Rojas M. Role of the SDF-1/CXCR4 axis in the pathogenesis of lung injury and fibrosis. Am J Respir Cell Mol Biol. 2007;37:291–9. doi:10.1165/rcmb.2006-0187OC.

43. Bundesmann MM, Wagner TE, Chow Y-H, Altemeier WA, Steinbach T, Schnapp LM. Role of urokinase plasminogen activator receptor-associated protein in mouse lung. Am J Respir Cell Mol Biol. 2012;46:233–9. doi:10.1165/rcmb.2010-0485OC.

44. Das S, MacDonald K, Chang H-YS, Mitzner W. A simple method of mouse lung intubation. J Vis Exp. 2013; e50318. doi:10.3791/50318.

45. Cai Y, Kimura S. Noninvasive intratracheal intubation to study the pathology and physiology of mouse lung. J Vis Exp. 2013; e50601. doi:10.3791/50601.

46. Thomas JL, Dumouchel J, Li J, Magat J, Balitzer D, Bigby TD. Endotracheal intubation in mice via direct laryngoscopy using an otoscope. J Vis Exp. 2014;. doi:10.3791/50269.

47. Ventilation with lower tidal volumes as compared with traditional tidal volumes for acute lung injury and the acute respiratory distress syndrome. The Acute Respiratory Distress Syndrome Network. N Engl J Med. 2000;342:1301–8. doi:10.1056/NEJM200005043421801.

48. O'Mahony DS, Liles WC, Altemeier WA, Dhanireddy S, Frevert CW, Liggitt D, et al. Mechanical ventilation interacts with endotoxemia to induce extrapulmonary organ dysfunction. Crit Care. 2006;10:R136. doi:10.1186/cc5050.

49. Gharib SA, Liles WC, Matute-Bello G, Glenny RW, Martin TR, Altemeier WA. Computational identification of key biological modules and transcription factors in acute lung injury. Am J Respir Crit Care Med. 2006;173:653–8. doi:10.1164/rccm.200509-1473OC.
50. Gharib SA, Liles WC, Klaff LS, Altemeier WA. Noninjurious mechanical ventilation activates a proinflammatory transcriptional program in the lung. Physiol Genomics. 2009;37:239–48. doi:10.1152/physiolgenomics.00027.2009.
51. Bomsztyk K, Mar D, An D, Sharifian R, Mikula M, Gharib SA, et al. Experimental acute lung injury induces multi-organ epigenetic modifications in key angiogenic genes implicated in sepsis-associated endothelial dysfunction. Crit Care. 2015;19:225. doi:10.1186/s13054-015-0943-4.
52. Gharib SA, Mar D, Bomsztyk K, Denisenko O, Dhanireddy S, Liles WC, et al. System-wide mapping of activated circuitry in experimental systemic inflammatory response syndrome. Shock. 2016;45:148–56. doi:10.1097/SHK.0000000000000507.
53. Oeckler RA, Lee W-Y, Park M-G, Kofler O, Rasmussen DL, Lee H-B, et al. Determinants of plasma membrane wounding by deforming stress. Am J Physiol Lung Cell Mol Physiol. 2010;299:L826–33. doi:10.1152/ajplung.00217.2010.
54. Plataki M, Lee YD, Rasmussen DL, Hubmayr RD. Poloxamer 188 facilitates the repair of alveolus resident cells in ventilator-injured lungs. Am J Respir Crit Care Med. 2011;184:939–47. doi:10.1164/rccm.201104-0647OC.
55. Hsia CCW, Hyde DM, Ochs M, Weibel ER, ATS/ERS Joint Task Force on Quantitative Assessment of Lung Structure. An official research policy statement of the American Thoracic Society/European Respiratory Society: standards for quantitative assessment of lung structure. Am J Respir Crit Care Med. 2010. p. 394–418. doi:10.1164/rccm.200809-1522ST.
56. Moitra J, Sammani S, Garcia JGN. Re-evaluation of Evans Blue dye as a marker of albumin clearance in murine models of acute lung injury. Transl Res. 2007;150:253–65. doi:10.1016/j.trsl.2007.03.013.
57. Bates JHT. Pulmonary mechanics: a system identification perspective. Conf Proc IEEE Eng Med Biol Soc. 2009;1:170–2. doi:10.1109/IEMBS.2009.5333302.
58. Foster WM, Walters DM, Longphre M, Macri K, Miller LM. Methodology for the measurement of mucociliary function in the mouse by scintigraphy. J Appl Physiol. 2001;90:1111–7.

Chapter 3
Transgenic Animal Models in Lung Research

Chi F. Hung and William A. Altemeier

Introduction

Advances in molecular biology have enabled the use of genetically modified mammalian vertebrates in human disease research. Due to their physiological similarity to humans, relative cost-effectiveness, and ease of husbandry, rodents have become the most widely used transgenic animals in modeling human disease. The goal of this chapter is not to undertake an exhaustive review of the history of transgenic animals, but rather to highlight recent advances in animal models used in pulmonary research and to offer practical guidance in the use of these transgenic animals. Over the past decade, the development of Cre-loxP technology has enabled the development of sophisticated transgenic animal models to address complex questions about development and function. While this technology is a powerful tool, many considerations need to be made when using these transgenic models. This chapter will give a brief overview of this technology as well as practical considerations in the use of these transgenic animals.

Transgenic Mice in Lung Injury Studies

Ever since the ability to introduce genetic modifications into mammalian embryonic stem cells was discovered in the 1980s, transgenic mice have assumed an integral role in the laboratory study of human disease [1]. Manipulations that result in

C.F. Hung (✉) · W.A. Altemeier
Division of Pulmonary and Critical Care Medicine, Department of Medicine,
Center for Lung Biology, University of Washington, Seattle, WA, USA
e-mail: cfhung@uw.edu

W.A. Altemeier
e-mail: billa@uw.edu

© Springer International Publishing AG 2017
L.M. Schnapp and C. Feghali-Bostwick (eds.), *Acute Lung Injury and Repair*,
Respiratory Medicine, DOI 10.1007/978-3-319-46527-2_3

gain-of-function and loss-of-function animal models have been used extensively over the last three decades to study biological pathways in lung pathogenesis. Heritable gene knock-ins and knockouts have been traditionally used to model human disease. Baron et al. [2] summarized genetically modified strains in their review of transgenic animals in lung biology research. For example, genetic knockouts of surfactant protein D and tissue inhibitor of metalloproteinases-3 lead to spontaneous histological changes compatible with chronic obstructive pulmonary disease [3, 4]. Models in which genetic manipulation does not lead to an overt phenotype but confers susceptibility to or protection against an injurious agent have also been widely used. For example, metalloproteinase-12 knockout mice have no observable lung phenotype during embryogenesis or in adulthood, however they are protected against emphysema with cigarette exposure [5]. These studies suggest metalloproteinases play a complex but important biological role airway inflammation, remodeling, and development of emphysematous changes.

Use of transgenic mice with global gene disruption has its limitations. Global knockout or overexpression of a gene may disrupt development and lead to embryonic or postnatal lethality. Conversely, biological pathways in pathogenesis may differ between species. Genetic manipulation in mice may not adequately recapitulate human disease. For example, attempts to generate a mouse model of alpha-1 antitrypsin (A1T1) deficiency have been unsuccessful to date. Depending on the mouse genetic background, serine protease expression in mice is controlled by multiple genes in the serpin family (Serpina1) whereas in humans, A1T1 expression is limited to one gene. Attempts to generate a knockout in one of the serine protease genes in mice (Serpina1a) have not been successful to date, with the unexpected discovery that Serpina1a-/- leads to embryonic lethality [6]. While human A1T1 expression is only controlled by one gene, Serpina1 null genotypes have been reported in humans suggesting A1T1 is not essential in human embryogenesis in contrast to mice. Given the important limitations seen in the generation of global knockout transgenic animals, other genetic manipulation strategies are required to study individual biological pathways in animal models. Recent advances in technologies that allow temporal and spatial control of genomic manipulation in mouse models are paving way to elegant transgenic models that address some of the limitations encountered in global knockout models.

Cre recombinase

Genomic manipulation using site-specific recombinases has become increasingly popular in transgenic mouse models. Recombinases are enzymes that serve a host of vital biological function in viruses and yeast. They recognize specific DNA sequences on the genome and mediate rearrangement of DNA with high efficiency, enabling molecular phenomena such as viral genomic integration and excision. The Cre recombinase derives from bacteriophage P1 and mediates recombination at specific 34 base pair sequences termed loxP sites [7, 8]. Of the many recombinases known, Cre recombinase requires no additional accessory proteins or specific substrate topology to mediate recombination efficiently at loxP sites [9, 10]. For these reasons, the Cre-loxP system has been widely used in transgenic mouse models to modify gene expression. Another well-studied recombinase with applications in transgenic animal studies includes the yeast recombinase Flp from *Saccharomyces cerevisiae* [11]. Application of these recombinases has enabled a host of novel studies in lung research including developmental studies, cell-fate mapping, and spatial or temporal gene disruption duties.

The 34 bp loxP sequence is directional. When two loxP sites are inserted into the host genome or linearized DNA in a head-to-tail fashion, Cre will mediate recombination between the loxP sites leading to the excision of the DNA between the loxP sites as a circular DNA plasmid [12]. In transgenic models, loxP sites may be introduced into targeted coding sequences in a specific gene (called a "floxed" gene). When crossed with a transgenic animal that expresses Cre recombinase under the control of a specific gene promoter, the bitransgenic progeny will undergo deletions of the floxed coding sequences where Cre recombinase is expressed. Such deletions may result in frameshift mutations or truncations during mRNA transcription, leading to null phenotypes.

Applications of Cre-loxP System in Animal Models

Studies in lung development and regeneration. The ability to manipulate the mouse genome using Cre-loxP transgenes was first demonstrated by Lewandoski and Martin [13] in 1997. The introduction of Cre-loxP technology in transgenic models has enabled a number of exciting discoveries and refinements in our understanding of cardiopulmonary development and regeneration. In these studies, transgenic animals expressing Cre under the control of a developmental gene promoter are crossed to transgenic animals carrying a reporter construct under the control of a ubiquitous promoter such as *Rosa26*. These constructs contain a STOP codon flanked by loxP sequences, and a chemical or fluorescent reporter downstream such as LacZ or any one of the fluorescent proteins (e.g., green fluorescent protein, tdTomato, yellow fluorescent protein) [14]. The result is constitutive silencing of the reporter until the floxed STOP codon is excised in the presence of Cre recombinase. In the presence of Cre recombinase, cells and their daughter cells constitutively and heritably express the reporter construct. Bitransgenic animals expressing Cre under a specific gene promoter (e.g., a gene of interest expressed only during embryonic development in a specific progenitor cell type) and the Rosa26-STOP$^{flox/flox}$-reporter transgene allow investigators to map the fate of early progenitor cells by visualizing labeled cells and their daughter cells in the developing lung. The ability to identify the temporal and spatial fate of lung progenitor cells allows for more detailed examination of the pathways essential to the proper differentiation of the many lung cell types and improved understanding of disease states. Similarly, whereas the fully developed adult lung remains fairly quiescent, adult progenitor populations are present and may reenter cell cycle to repair and/or regenerate damaged cells following experimental injury stimuli. While the composition of and pathways utilized by these putative adult progenitor cells remain unclear, Cre-loxP technology has enabled a number of studies directed at identification of the pools of progenitor cells in the adult lung. For example, labeling of differentiated type II alveolar epithelial cells has shown that they are capable of acting as stem cells to repair damaged alveolar epithelium following lung injury [15]. Furthermore, this technology has been used to identify the progenitors of lung myofibroblasts following experimental lung injury and to expand on the field's understanding of the key cellular effectors in fibrosis and lung repair [16, 17].

Spatial deletions. Another powerful application of Cre-loxP technology is its use in cell-specific deletion of genes. By carefully selecting cell type-specific promoters, investigators are able to engineer transgenic mice with targeted gene deletions in restricted populations of lung cells. These studies have led to a more refined understanding of the functional heterogeneity of different cell types in lung injury and repair. For example, an area of intense debate within the lung fibrosis field has been whether bone-marrow-derived, circulating progenitor cells termed "fibrocytes" directly contribute to collagen I deposition in lung fibrosis. These cells are CD45+ and display collagen $I\alpha I$ gene and protein expression. Furthermore, they localized to areas of fibrosis in experimental models of lung injury by immunohistochemistry [18] However, conflicting data have shown no evidence of CD45+ cells in areas of fibrosis by lineage-tracing studies [16, 17], calling into question the importance of fibrocytes in lung fibrosis. Kleaveland et al. further elaborated on these findings and examined collagen I production by fibrocytes in experimental lung injury. In their study, transgenic mice expressing Cre under a hematopoietic cell lineage promoter, Vav-Cre, crossed to a *collagen $I\alpha I$* floxed transgenic animal were used to disrupt *collagen $I\alpha I$* expression specifically in fibrocytes, without affecting fibrogenic cell types of non-hematopoietic lineages. Despite the inability of fibrocytes to transcribe the *collagen $I\alpha I$* gene, collagen I deposition was unaffected in experimentally induced lung fibrosis. Therefore, the authors concluded fibrocytes did not functionally contribute to collagen I deposition [19]. Without the ability to restrict the deletion of the *collagen $I\alpha I$* gene in fibrocytes, this type of study would not be possible. Another advantage of spatial deletion in gene disruption studies is that global knockout of a gene of interest sometimes leads to an embryonic lethal phenotype, rendering the model unsuitable for studies requiring adult animals.

Temporal Cre activation and deletions. A related application of the Cre-LoxP system involves the conditional activation of Cre in a temporally controlled manner. To achieve this, various constructs of Cre recombinase fused to ligand-binding domains have been generated, resulting in Cre recombinase (tethered to a ligand-binding domain) that is sequestered in the cytosolic compartment and unable to mediate genomic recombination at target loxP sites. Upon ligand exposure and binding to the ligand-binding domain (typically exogenously administered at the desired time point), Cre recombinase translocates to the nucleus to mediate genomic recombination. The most commonly used conditionally activated Cre recombinases involve mutated estrogen receptors and the administration of tamoxifen to liberate the Cre recombinases. Various widely available constructs include CreER, CreER^{T2}, and MerCreMer. The ability to temporally control Cre activation enables studies in which timed recombination of the target, floxed gene is desired. For example, conditional knockout of a gene critical in development can be studied in adults using the CreER technology by administering tamoxifen to adults, thus bypassing the developmental stage where the gene's function is vital.

Inducible Cre beyond tamoxifen. The doxycycline system was developed to reversibly suppress or activate gene expression in transgenic mice. This transgenic model consists of two transgenic lines bred to each other: (1) an activator line expressing either the tetracycline activator (TA, or tet-off) or the reverse tetracycline responsive transactivator (rtTA, or tet-on) and (2) an operator line with the desired transgene under the control of the tetO operator. In bitransgenic animals containing the activator and operator transgenes, doxycycline administration allows tetracycline activator to bind to tetO, suppressing transgene expression downstream (tet-off), or rtTA to bind to tetO, activating transgene expression (tet-on). This model was developed separately from the Cre/lox model to study gene expression in mouse models. Combining the Cre/lox system with tetO system has allowed for sophisticated methodolgies in doxycycline-dependent, cre-mediated gene manipulations. The generation of triple transgenic mice with rtTA expression under a cell-specific promoter, TetO-Cre, and loxP sites flanking a gene of interest result in animals that will have deletion of a gene of interest in a cell-specific manner when they are exposed to a diet with doxycycline. Perl et al. used this strategy to generate a triple transgenic animal combining rtTA expression under the SP-C promoter for epithelial tissue specificity, tetO-Cre, and CMV-loxP-LacZ-loxP-AP (ZAP) or CMV-loxP-LacZ-loxP-GFP (ZEG) reporter construct [20]. Following doxycycline exposure, these mice demonstrated reporter expression (alkaline phosphatase or GFP) in distal lung epithelial cells.

In addition to doxycycline, other inducers have been described. The use of a Cre fused to a progesterone receptor ligand-binding domain was first described by Kellendonk et al. [21]. In these transgenic mice, Cre activity is induced by the administration of RU-486. However, transgenic mice using this fusion Cre showed variable "leaky Cre" activity in which Cre activity was observed in unexposed transgenic animals (i.e., no RU-486) [22, 23]. Partly due to the leaky Cre phenomenon, inducible Cre transgenic lines using progesterone receptor ligand-binding domain fusion are less widely available compared to the tamoxifen-inducible CreER or CreER^{T2} counterparts.

Novel inducible Cre lines are under development to harness advances in pharmacologic stabilization of destabilized proteins. This technology utilizes mutant destabilizing proteins from humans or bacteria fused to a protein of interest. When the protein of interest is fused to the destabilizing protein, the complex is usually degraded by proteosomes. However, this degradation can be blocked by administration of a pharmacologic stabilizing agent. For example, Cre recombinase has been fused with the destabilizing dihydrofolate reductase (DHFR) from *Escherichia coli* to generate an inducible Cre transgenic animal that targets genes specifically in neurons [24]. In this model, the administration of trimethoprim (TMX) stabilizes the Cre-DHFR fusion protein driven by a neuron-specific promoter and leads to efficient Cre-mediated recombination in neurons. The advantage of TMX-inducible system includes ease of administration in animal models, high penetrance in most tissues, and lack of endogenous targets in mammals. This may prove to be a highly attractive model in lung research, but specific transgenic lines have yet to be developed and characterized for lung biology.

Lung-specific Cre Mouse Models

Murine lung derives from the endoderm foregut and develops by branching morphogenesis. Differentiation of various lung cell types appears during lung development. A number of transgenic models using lung-specific and nonspecific promoters to drive Cre expression have been developed to examine the fate and function of various progenitors and differentiated lung cell populations. Lung bud from the foregut appears around E9.5 in mice while the trachea and esophagus separate from the foregut between E10.0 and E11.5. The choice of transgenic model and timing of inducible Cre activity will influence the lung specificity of the model.

Lung epithelium. Models for epithelial progenitors, type II alveolar epithelial cells (ATII), type I alveolar epithelial cells (ATI), Clara cells, basal cells, and ciliated cells have been developed. The human surfactant associated protein C (Sftpc) promoter has been used to generate transgenic strains that specifically target the lung epithelium. In the developed, adult lung, Sftpc promoter expression is restricted to ATII and some cuboidal bronchiolar cells. During embryogenesis, however, the promoter is active once the endoderm is committed to lung development and drives recombination throughout the lung epithelium [25]. Another transgenic line Sftpc-CreERt2-rtTA has been developed that contains a knock-in of the CreERt2 and rtTA cassettes in the endogenous mouse Sftpc promoter [26]. Expression of CreERt2 and rtTA in this line is restricted to ATII cells in the adult lung and may present a very useful model to examine conditional gene disruption in ATII cells.

Still other Cre transgenic mice are available to study lung epithelial cells though they are not lung specific. Transgenic models that utilize promoters active in epithelial precursor cells are active in the endoderm before lung bud formation, and thus may drive expression in extrapulmonary tissues following embryogenesis. Sonic hedgehog (Shh) knock-in Cre-GFP is active in the ventral foregut endoderm by E9.5 before lung and trachea-esophagus separation. Islet1-Cre is a knock-in Cre line with expression in pharyngeal endoderm by E9.5. While it labels the lung epithelial precursor cells widely, it is not specific to the lung epithelium. Small populations of mesenchyme are also labeled by this strain. The Id2-CreERt2 is a CreERt2 knock-in mice that shows tamoxifen-dependent activity in distal epithelial tips and a subset of mesenchymal cells. Nkx2-5 Cre is another knock-in transgenic line that has been used to disrupt lung epithelial genes, however Nkx2-5 is also active throughout the foregut endoderm and the surrounding mesoderm before lung budding, and thus has activity in other developing organs such as the myocardium as well [27].

While transgenic mice using the Sftpc promoter to label ATII cells are fairly specific to the lungs, promoters for ATI cells are less specific. Aquaporin 5 (Aqp5) is expressed in ATI but not ATII cells in rats and humans. Mice express Aqp5 predominantly in ATI cells and in a small minority of ATII cells. Cre transgenic mice using the Aqp5 promoter have been developed but extrapulmonary expression (e.g., salivary glands and stomach) has also been observed [28]. To date, no transgenic line exists with Cre activity exclusively in ATI cells.

Lung stromal cells. Stromal cells in the lung have traditionally been defined by negatives: they are non-epithelial, non-endothelial, and non-immune. These interstitial cells are histologically and functionally heterogeneous with potentially very different roles in lung pathobiology. Contractile smooth muscles that surround larger airways and arterioles constitute one type of stromal cell. Perivascular stromal cells at the capillary level (also termed pericytes) constitute a histologically and functionally distinct subtype of stromal cell. Finally, interstitial fibroblasts in alveoli may constitute yet another functionally distinct group of stromal cells. Within the group of fibroblasts, there are further functional and histological distinctions such as lipofibroblasts and matrix-producing fibroblasts. Classification of stromal subpopulations remains controversial and there is no consensus on markers that uniquely identify each of these stromal cell subtypes. Exactly how these cellular subtypes contribute to lung repair remains under active investigation. For example, recent studies using lineage-tracing mouse models have shown that multiple stromal populations including resident fibroblasts and pericytes contribute to scar-forming cells in experimental lung fibrosis [16, 17]. To understand the function and lineages of the diverse populations of stromal cells, investigators have developed transgenic Cre models that trace the lineage of various mesenchymal cell types, though none of the models is specific to the lung. We have used a mouse model originally developed to fate-trace pericyte progenitors in the kidney and examined its suitability as a pericyte lineage-tracing model in the adult mouse lung [29]. FoxD1 is a forkhead transcription factor expressed only during embryonic development. We observed that FoxD1-derived cells are enriched for platelet-derived growth factor receptor beta positive stromal cells in the adult mouse lung and are histologically compatible with pericytes [16]. The FoxD1-Cre model thus represents a useful tool for examining the function of pericytes in the lung. To study smooth muscle cells, various transgenic Cre models utilizing promoters SM22α, smooth muscle actin α (SMA), and smooth muscle myosin heavy chain (SMMHC) have been developed [30]. Their utility in the adult mouse lung is limited by the fact that Cre activity is not inducible in these lines. Inducible Cre lines using the SMA and SMMHC promoters have been developed and these lines may prove to be useful tools in studying smooth muscle and myofibroblast function in the adult mouse lung [31, 32].

Lung endothelial cells. To date, there is no lung-specific endothelial transgenic mouse line. The most widely used endothelial lineage-tracing model utilizes the murine Tek promoter (commonly referred to as Tie2) [33]. Tie2-Cre mice labels endothelial cells in many organs and have been a useful tool in vascular biology research. The utility of this model in lung biology is limited by its widespread expression throughout the mouse vasculature and caution must be made when using this line as nonspecific activity, presumably transmitted through germline activation of Cre, has been reported [34]. Individuals with an interest in lung-specific Cre transgenic lines are encouraged to read a comprehensive review on this topic by Rawlins and Perl [35].

Protocols

Tamoxifen preparation. Numerous resources and protocols are available online for the preparation of tamoxifen. Tamoxifen is a hydrophobic compound and thus dissolves poorly in aqueous solutions. Most commonly, tamoxifen is supplied in powder form and needs to be reconstituted fresh prior to each administration. Tamoxifen is soluble in ethanol, methanol, 2-propanol, and propylene glycol. Common preparations of injectable tamoxifen involve dissolving tamoxifen powder (Sigma T5648) in ethanol (commonly to a final concentration of 50 mg/ml). Preheating the ethanol to 37 °C aids in solubilizing the tamoxifen powder. Aliquots of tamoxifen prepared in this manner may be stored in −20 °C for several months but should be kept from light exposure. Prior to injection, aliquots are further diluted in 4× volume of corn oil (Sigma C8267) and then injected into the peritoneum of animals. Concentrations of tamoxifen greater than 10–20 mg/ml in corn oil may result in tamoxifen becoming insoluble and precipitating out of solution. A typical preparation includes dissolving tamoxifen powder in 100 % ethanol to a stock concentration of 50 mg/ml. Prior to injection, the stock solution is further diluted in 4× volume of corn oil to a concentration of 10 mg/ml. Injection of 100 µl of tamoxifen in corn oil (10 mg/ml, or 1 mg per injection) may be adequate to activate the recombinase. Users are advised to consult with IACUC at their institutions to determine an appropriate injection schedule and the maximum allowable dosage. One disadvantage we observed with this method is that mice (C57bl6 background) may have poor absorption of the corn oil solution. At necropsy 4–5 weeks beyond the last administration of tamoxifen, oil droplets may continue to be present in the peritoneum. Furthermore, studding of the diaphragm and peritoneum with white plaques has been observed by many investigators which may represent insoluble tamoxifen deposits or from the corn oil. To address these concerns, alternative vehicles to emulsify poorly water-soluble tamoxifen have been tested. Kolliphor (previously Cremophor) is an amphiphilic polyethoxylated castor oil derivative that is commonly used to solubilize poorly water-soluble pharmacologic agents. It has been used to solubilize tamoxifen for intraperitoneal as well as intravenous injection of tamoxifen [36]:

- Add prewarmed 100 % ethanol (37 °C) to dissolve tamoxifen powder (conc. 50 mg/ml)
- Vortex to dissolve tamoxifen completely (usually 5–10 min is adequate)
- Add equal volume of Kolliphor (Sigma C5135) to tamoxifen/ethanol mix (tamoxifen conc. 25 mg/ml)
- Vortex and mix well. Aliquot and store in −20 °C protected from light
- To use: add 4× volume of PBS to Kolliphor/tamoxifen/ethanol mix and vortex well to ensure complete emulsification (final tamoxifen conc. 5 mg/ml). For 1 mg tamoxifen administrations, use 200 µl.

Tamoxifen administration. Tamoxifen may be administered by various routes. The most common route of administration is by intraperitoneal injection. Commonly, injection schedules of one to five times once daily are performed depending on the efficiency of Cre-mediated recombination. Intravenous administration using the Kolliphor preparation emulsified in sterile saline has also been reported [36].

For schedules that require multiple daily injections, the labor required presents a major disadvantage. Moreover, multiple injections increase the stress experienced by animals and the risk of organ injury during injections. A less labor-intensive alternative that is equally effective is by feeding tamoxifen-impregnated pellet food. A number of vendors have made these pellet feeds widely commercially available but care must be taken to ensure the animals are accepting the pellet food when it is first introduced. Various strategies to help the animals acclimate to the tamoxifen chow exist and they include: addition of sucrose to the pellet (can be done by the vendor), wetting the food in the initial stages, and introducing the tamoxifen chow mixed with regular chow in the beginning. Consultation with veterinary services responsible for care of animals at the research facility prior to initiation of tamoxifen feed is essential to develop monitoring and action plans for the period when mice are placed on special diet.

Special Considerations (Troubleshooting)

Tissue-dependent efficiency. The efficiencies of Cre recombinase expression as well as Cre-mediated recombination at loxP sites are dependent on the promoter driving the Cre expression, the level of Cre recombinase activity in the cell, the location and distance of loxP sites, and the tissue in which recombination occurs [37–39]. A number of observations from published reports suggest Cre expression may not be uniform between organs despite the use of a universal promoter. For instance, the ubiquitous strain CAGGCreER[TM] has a widespread expression of CreER and administration of tamoxifen to either pregnant dams or adult mice induces widespread Cre-mediated recombination [40]. However, multiple observations show that penetrance of Cre activity is dose dependent, and importantly, some organs show incomplete Cre activity despite high doses of tamoxifen [40]. To ensure the proper expression of Cre, investigators must characterize the specificity of Cre activity in the organ or cell type of interest with a reporter line before developing Cre/lox animals in gene deletion studies.

Cre toxicity. The presence of Cre recombinase alone may lead to cellular toxicity. Observations in Cre transgenic animals have shown that Cre recombinase may have various cytotoxic effects. First, sites that mimic loxP sequences exist in the mammalian genome and they may serve as unintended targets of Cre recombinase in transgenic animals even in the absence of loxP sites [41, 42]. Such off-target activity may lead to unintended DNA damage and/or rearrangement, a phenomenon that has been observed in transgenic mice [43, 44]. Second, Cre recombinase itself may act as a transcriptional repressor. As the recombination product between two loxP sites leaves one loxP site on the genomic DNA and one loxP site on the excised fragment, continued production of Cre recombinase in the cell may lead to Cre recombinase occupying the recombined loxP sequence on the genomic DNA. This event has the potential to inhibit transcription downstream from the occupied loxP sequence [45]. Third, lessons from cardiovascular research suggest phenotypic alterations may result in transgenic animals due solely to the presence of Cre recombinase. Use of α-myosin heavy chain (aMHC) gene as a cardiomyocyte-specific promoter for Cre recombinase has been extensively studied in cardiovascular literature. The tamoxifen-sensitive aMHC-MerCreMer transgenic mice have been observed to develop cardiac dysfunction independent of side effects from tamoxifen exposure or intended gene disruption in aMHC-MerCreMer myocytes. Phenotypes ranging from cardiac fibrosis to dilated cardiomyopathy have been observed in these transgenic mice [46–48]. Inclusion of Cre transgenic animals without the loxP transgene as controls is thus recommended in studies where the experimental endpoint may be affected by Cre toxicity.

Parental Cre transmission. Another factor to consider when breeding Cre transgenic animals for lineage or gene disruption studies is the choice of parents carrying the Cre transgene. Whether Cre is maternally or paternally transmitted may have a significant impact on the phenotype of the offspring. It has been observed that Cre activity may be more active in the offspring depending on whether the Cre transgene is transmitted through the mother or the father. For example, the EIIa-Cre transgenic mouse displays widespread Cre activity in all tissues when the EIIa-Cre transgene is transmitted maternally. In contrast, the EIIa-Cre transgene activity is spatially mosaic and sparse when transmitted paternally [49]. This difference could be explained by the post-zygotic persistence of Cre activity expressed in the maternal germline. Cam2a-Cre, which is designed to restrict Cre expression to the hippocampus, demonstrates Cre expression in the male germ line cells (http://cre.jax.org/Camk2a/Camk2a-creNano.html) as well. In our own experience with the FoxD1-Cre line, we have found the parental transmission to be an integral part of experimental design. FoxD1 encodes a forkhead transcription factor that is active during embryonic development and is subsequently silenced in the adult mouse. The lineage of mesenchymal cells that express FoxD1 during development labels perivascular stromal cells (or pericytes) in the adult kidney and lung [16]. When a FoxD1-Cre;Rosa26-floxSTOP-tdTomato male breeder is used, we found in certain offspring widespread expression of the tdTomato reporter, even in the absence of the Cre transgene. This was likely a result of Cre activity in the male germline that passed on the recombined reporter transgene to the offspring. Thus, we adjusted the breeding strategy when using this line such that the breeder female carries the FoxD1-Cre trangene to minimize the effect of male germline Cre activity. Therefore, depending on the promoter driving Cre expression, consideration for parental transmission must be made and generation of reporter animals to examine tissue/cell-type specificity of Cre activity in the offspring is often a necessary first step prior to carrying out further experiments.

Leaky inducible Cre. For certain genes, generation of knockout transgenic mice may lead to undesired or unexpected phenotypes, such as embryonic lethality or aberrant development. The ability to temporally control the gene deletion or modification through conditional knockouts models is thus an essential part of working with transgenic animals. The advent of inducible Cre lines has become a powerful tool in this regard. While inducible Cre constructs are designed to exclude Cre recombinase from the nucleus until ligand binding (e.g., tamoxifen administration in Cre-ERT transgenic mice), there are reports of Cre activity in the absence of ligand administration. This phenomenon has been termed "leaky Cre." One example of leaky Cre is seen in the RIP-CreER transgenic line. RIP is a rat insulin promoter expressed in insulin-producing pancreatic beta islet cells. This transgenic line has been used to study the origin of beta cells in mice. However, RIP-CreER transgenic mice can display Cre recombinase activity as early as 2 months of age even in the absence of tamoxifen exposure [50]. The phenomenon highlights the importance of validating the inducible Cre transgenic line by crossing with a reporter such as Rosa26-lacZ or Rosa26-tdTomato to look for evidence of autonomous Cre activity in the absence of inducer.

Cre mosaicism and incomplete recombination. Different tissues and different genes allow varying efficiencies in Cre-mediated recombination. Ubiquitous promoters that drive conditional CreER expression may display varying degrees of Cre recombinase activity depending on the tissue. Examples of this can be seen at the Jackson Laboratory website with the chicken beta-actin promoter (http://cre.jax.org/Cag-creERT/Cag-creESR1.html) or the human ubiquitin C promoter (http://cre.jax.org/UBC-creERT/UBC-creERT.html). In addition to tissue dependence, efficiency of recombination is also dependent on the gene being targeted. Voojis et al. showed that inducible Cre recombinase activity varies not only between tissues but also between different genes using a Rosa26-CreERT transgenic animal with Rb flox, p53 flox, and Brca2 flox transgenes [39]. When using Cre or inducible Cre to delete genes, it is therefore important to ensure the gene of interest does in fact undergo efficient recombination in the organ of interest.

Controls. Given the numerous unintended consequences that may be introduced with Cre transgene expression, it is important to design animal experiments with the appropriate controls. Littermates without Cre expression are standardly used as controls alongside experimental animals with Cre expression. Mice with Cre expression but without the floxed genes may serve as additional controls if there is evidence that Cre expression under the specific promoter leads to phenotypic alteration in animals, as is the case with aMHC-MerCreMer mice discussed previously. Confirmation that the intended gene product is deleted at the protein level (preferred) or by genomic DNA analysis in experimental animals is important to ensure valid interpretation of experimental results.

References

1. Manis JP. Knock out, knock in, knock down–genetically manipulated mice and the Nobel Prize. N Engl J Med. 2007;357(24):2426–9.
2. Baron RM, Choi AJ, Owen CA, Choi AM. Genetically manipulated mouse models of lung disease: potential and pitfalls. Am J Physiol Lung Cell Mol Physiol. 2012;302(6):L485–97.
3. Yoshida M, Korfhagen TR, Whitsett JA. Surfactant protein D regulates NF-kappa B and matrix metalloproteinase production in alveolar macrophages via oxidant-sensitive pathways. J Immunol. 2001;166(12):7514–9.
4. Leco KJ, Waterhouse P, Sanchez OH, Gowing KL, Poole AR, Wakeham A, Mak TW, Khokha R. Spontaneous air space enlargement in the lungs of mice lacking tissue inhibitor of metalloproteinases-3 (TIMP-3). J Clin Investig. 2001;108(6):817–29.
5. Hautamaki RD, Kobayashi DK, Senior RM, Shapiro SD. Requirement for macrophage elastase for cigarette smoke-induced emphysema in mice. Science. 1997;277(5334):2002–4.
6. Wang D, Wang W, Dawkins P, Paterson T, Kalsheker N, Sallenave JM, Houghton AM. Deletion of Serpina1a, a murine alpha1-antitrypsin ortholog, results in embryonic lethality. Exp Lung Res. 2011;37(5):291–300.
7. Sternberg N, Hamilton D. Bacteriophage P1 site-specific recombination. I. Recombination between loxP sites. J Mol Biol. 1981;150(4):467–86.
8. Sternberg N, Hamilton D, Hoess R. Bacteriophage P1 site-specific recombination. II. Recombination between loxP and the bacterial chromosome. J Mol Biol. 1981;150 (4):487–507.
9. Abremski K, Hoess R. Phage P1 Cre-loxP site-specific recombination. Effects of DNA supercoiling on catenation and knotting of recombinant products. J Mol Biol. 1985;184 (2):211–20.
10. Abremski K, Wierzbicki A, Frommer B, Hoess RH. Bacteriophage P1 Cre-loxP site-specific recombination. Site-specific DNA topoisomerase activity of the Cre recombination protein. J Biol Chem. 1986;261(1):391–6.
11. O'Gorman S, Fox DT, Wahl GM. Recombinase-mediated gene activation and site-specific integration in mammalian cells. Science. 1991;251(4999):1351–5.
12. Ghosh K, Van Duyne GD. Cre-loxP biochemistry. Methods. 2002;28(3):374–83.
13. Lewandoski M, Martin GR. Cre-mediated chromosome loss in mice. Nat Genet. 1997;17 (2):223–5.
14. Soriano P. Generalized lacZ expression with the ROSA26 Cre reporter strain. Nat Genet. 1999;21(1):70–1.
15. Barkauskas CE, Cronce MJ, Rackley CR, Bowie EJ, Keene DR, Stripp BR, Randell SH, Noble PW, Hogan BL. Type 2 alveolar cells are stem cells in adult lung. J Clin Investig. 2013;123(7):3025–36.
16. Hung C, Linn G, Chow YH, Kobayashi A, Mittelsteadt K, Altemeier WA, Gharib SA, Schnapp LM, Duffield JS. Role of lung pericytes and resident fibroblasts in the pathogenesis of pulmonary fibrosis. Am J Respir Crit Care Med. 2013;188(7):820–30.
17. Rock JR, Barkauskas CE, Cronce MJ, Xue Y, Harris JR, Liang J, Noble PW, Hogan BL. Multiple stromal populations contribute to pulmonary fibrosis without evidence for epithelial to mesenchymal transition. Proc Natl Acad Sci USA. 2011;108(52):E1475–83.

18. Phillips RJ, Burdick MD, Hong K, Lutz MA, Murray LA, Xue YY, Belperio JA, Keane MP, Strieter RM. Circulating fibrocytes traffic to the lungs in response to CXCL12 and mediate fibrosis. J Clin Investig. 2004;114(3):438–46.

19. Kleaveland KR, Velikoff M, Yang J, Agarwal M, Rippe RA, Moore BB, Kim KK. Fibrocytes are not an essential source of type I collagen during lung fibrosis. J Immunol. 2014;193 (10):5229–39.

20. Perl AK, Wert SE, Nagy A, Lobe CG, Whitsett JA. Early restriction of peripheral and proximal cell lineages during formation of the lung. Proc Natl Acad Sci USA. 2002;99 (16):10482–7.

21. Kellendonk C, Tronche F, Monaghan AP, Angrand PO, Stewart F, Schutz G. Regulation of Cre recombinase activity by the synthetic steroid RU 486. Nucleic Acids Res. 1996;24 (8):1404–11.

22. Kellendonk C, Tronche F, Casanova E, Anlag K, Opherk C, Schutz G. Inducible site-specific recombination in the brain. J Mol Biol. 1999;285(1):175–82.

23. Minamino T, Gaussin V, DeMayo FJ, Schneider MD. Inducible gene targeting in postnatal myocardium by cardiac-specific expression of a hormone-activated Cre fusion protein. Circ Res. 2001;88(6):587–92.

24. Sando R 3rd, Baumgaertel K, Pieraut S, Torabi-Rander N, Wandless TJ, Mayford M, Maximov A. Inducible control of gene expression with destabilized Cre. Nat Methods. 2013;10(11):1085–8.

25. Okubo T, Knoepfler PS, Eisenman RN, Hogan BL. Nmyc plays an essential role during lung development as a dosage-sensitive regulator of progenitor cell proliferation and differentiation. Development. 2005;132(6):1363–74.

26. Chapman HA, Li X, Alexander JP, Brumwell A, Lorizio W, Tan K, Sonnenberg A, Wei Y, Vu TH. Integrin alpha6beta4 identifies an adult distal lung epithelial population with regenerative potential in mice. J Clin Investig. 2011;121(7):2855–62.

27. Que J, Luo X, Schwartz RJ, Hogan BL. Multiple roles for Sox2 in the developing and adult mouse trachea. Development. 2009;136(11):1899–907.

28. Flodby P, Borok Z, Banfalvi A, Zhou B, Gao D, Minoo P, Ann DK, Morrisey EE, Crandall ED. Directed expression of Cre in alveolar epithelial type 1 cells. Am J Respir Cell Mol Biol. 2010;43(2):173–8.

29. Humphreys BD, Lin SL, Kobayashi A, Hudson TE, Nowlin BT, Bonventre JV, Valerius MT, McMahon AP, Duffield JS. Fate tracing reveals the pericyte and not epithelial origin of myofibroblasts in kidney fibrosis. Am J Pathol. 2010;176(1):85–97.

30. Wamhoff BR, Sinha S, Owens GK. Conditional mouse models to study developmental and pathophysiological gene function in muscle. Handb Exp Pharmacol. 2007;178:441–68.

31. Wendling O, Bornert JM, Chambon P, Metzger D. Efficient temporally-controlled targeted mutagenesis in smooth muscle cells of the adult mouse. Genesis. 2009;47(1):14–8.

32. Wirth A, Benyo Z, Lukasova M, Leutgeb B, Wettschureck N, Gorbey S, Orsy P, Horvath B, Maser-Gluth C, Greiner E, et al. G12-G13-LARG-mediated signaling in vascular smooth muscle is required for salt-induced hypertension. Nat Med. 2008;14(1):64–8.

33. Kisanuki YY, Hammer RE, Miyazaki J, Williams SC, Richardson JA, Yanagisawa M. Tie2-Cre transgenic mice: a new model for endothelial cell-lineage analysis in vivo. Dev Biol. 2001;230(2):230–42.

34. de Lange WJ, Halabi CM, Beyer AM, Sigmund CD. Germ line activation of the Tie2 and SMMHC promoters causes noncell-specific deletion of floxed alleles. Physiol Genomics. 2008;35(1):1–4.

35. Rawlins EL, Perl AK. The a"MAZE"ing world of lung-specific transgenic mice. Am J Respir Cell Mol Biol. 2012;46(3):269–82.

36. Chevalier C, Nicolas JF, Petit AC. Preparation and delivery of 4-hydroxy-tamoxifen for clonal and polyclonal labeling of cells of the surface ectoderm, skin, and hair follicle. Methods Mol Biol. 2014;1195:239–45.

37. Comai G, Sambasivan R, Gopalakrishnan S, Tajbakhsh S. Variations in the efficiency of lineage marking and ablation confound distinctions between myogenic cell populations. Dev Cell. 2014;31(5):654–67.
38. Lewandoski M. Conditional control of gene expression in the mouse. Nat Rev Genet. 2001;2 (10):743–55.
39. Vooijs M, Jonkers J, Berns A. A highly efficient ligand-regulated Cre recombinase mouse line shows that LoxP recombination is position dependent. EMBO Rep. 2001;2(4):292–7.
40. Hayashi S, McMahon AP. Efficient recombination in diverse tissues by a tamoxifen-inducible form of Cre: a tool for temporally regulated gene activation/inactivation in the mouse. Dev Biol. 2002;244(2):305–18.
41. Thyagarajan B, Guimaraes MJ, Groth AC, Calos MP. Mammalian genomes contain active recombinase recognition sites. Gene. 2000;244(1–2):47–54.
42. Ito M, Yamanouchi K, Naito K, Calos MP, Tojo H. Site-specific integration of transgene targeting an endogenous lox-like site in early mouse embryos. J Appl Genet. 2011;52 (1):89–94.
43. Janbandhu VC, Moik D, Fassler R. Cre recombinase induces DNA damage and tetraploidy in the absence of loxP sites. Cell Cycle. 2014;13(3):462–70.
44. Schmidt EE, Taylor DS, Prigge JR, Barnett S, Capecchi MR. Illegitimate Cre-dependent chromosome rearrangements in transgenic mouse spermatids. Proc Natl Acad Sci USA. 2000;97(25):13702–7.
45. Iovino N, Denti MA, Bozzoni I, Cortese R. A loxP-containing pol II promoter for RNA interference is reversibly regulated by Cre recombinase. RNA Biol. 2005;2(3):86–92.
46. Lexow J, Poggioli T, Sarathchandra P, Santini MP, Rosenthal N. Cardiac fibrosis in mice expressing an inducible myocardial-specific Cre driver. Dis Model Mech. 2013;6(6):1470–6.
47. Buerger A, Rozhitskaya O, Sherwood MC, Dorfman AL, Bisping E, Abel ED, Pu WT, Izumo S, Jay PY. Dilated cardiomyopathy resulting from high-level myocardial expression of Cre-recombinase. J Card Fail. 2006;12(5):392–8.
48. Koitabashi N, Bedja D, Zaiman AL, Pinto YM, Zhang M, Gabrielson KL, Takimoto E, Kass DA. Avoidance of transient cardiomyopathy in cardiomyocyte-targeted tamoxifen-induced MerCreMer gene deletion models. Circ Res. 2009;105(1):12–5.
49. Heffner CS, Herbert Pratt C, Babiuk RP, Sharma Y, Rockwood SF, Donahue LR, Eppig JT, Murray SA. Supporting conditional mouse mutagenesis with a comprehensive cre characterization resource. Nat Commun. 2012;3:1218.
50. Liu Y, Suckale J, Masjkur J, Magro MG, Steffen A, Anastassiadis K, Solimena M. Tamoxifen-Independent Recombination in the RIP-CreER Mouse. PLoS ONE. 2010;5(10): e13533.

Chapter 4
Fundamental Methods for Analysis of Acute Lung Injury in Mice

Carole L. Wilson, Lindsey M. Felton and Yu-Hua Chow

Introduction

The laboratory mouse has undoubtedly been an invaluable experimental tool for modeling acute lung injury (ALI) and pulmonary fibrosis. Several features of this mammal, including its small size (relatively inexpensive to house and easy to handle), rapid life cycle, and genetic malleability, make it close to ideal for studying mechanisms of lung injury and repair, despite there being some key physiological and anatomical differences between mouse and human respiratory systems [9, 10, 16]. Our intent in this chapter is to highlight some of the standard methods currently in practice to assess ALI in mice. A recent report from an American Thoracic Society (ATS) Workshop, which was tasked with obtaining a general consensus from leaders in the field on defining and measuring ALI in animal models, provides an excellent guide to the new (and seasoned) investigator in pulmonary biology on choosing injury models and methods of analysis [8]. The reader is also referred to several comprehensive, in-depth reviews that discuss other, more specialized methods to assess lung injury, particularly alveolar permeability and fluid clearance, as well as edema, in rodents [7, 12, 13].

The specific investigational avenues that are taken to analyze ALI in mice depend on several factors, including the experimental questions being asked, the

C.L. Wilson (✉) · L.M. Felton
Division of Pulmonary, Critical Care, Allergy, and Sleep Medicine, Medical University of South Carolina, 96 Jonathan Lucas Street, MSC 630, Charleston, SC 29425, USA
e-mail: wilsocar@musc.edu

L.M. Felton
e-mail: felton@musc.edu

Y.-H. Chow
Division of Pulmonary and Cricial Care Medicine, University of Washington School of Medicine, 850 Republican Street, Seattle, WA 98109, USA
e-mail: chowy@uw.edu

© Springer International Publishing AG 2017
L.M. Schnapp and C. Feghali-Bostwick (eds.), *Acute Lung Injury and Repair*,
Respiratory Medicine, DOI 10.1007/978-3-319-46527-2_4

pertinent aspects of ALI being evaluated, and the feasibility and practicality of obtaining the desired measurements. The four major outcomes of ALI in mice include (1) disruption of the alveolar capillary barrier, (2) histopathological changes in lung architecture, (3) localized inflammation, and (4) physiological dysfunction, with (1) and (2) considered the most relevant features. The ATS Workshop suggested that at least three of these four features should be analyzed to definitively establish that ALI has occurred in animal models, with the caveat that some experimental objectives may not require that all ALI features be present [8]. In the following sections of this chapter, we will outline and describe in detail the basic methods we use in our laboratory to address parameters 1–3 listed above. Note that some methods allow assessment of more than one feature of ALI. An approach to analyze physiological dysfunction by measuring lung mechanics is covered in a separate chapter in this book.

Bronchoalveolar Lavage

Bronchoalveolar lavage (BAL) is a key tool for sampling the secretions and loosely attached cells of the peripheral airways and alveoli. This versatile technique allows the investigator to obtain quantitative measures of the extent of inflammation and changes in permeability in the injured lung (two of the four ALI parameters). Although BAL can theoretically be performed multiple times in anesthetized mice and can be targeted to specific lobes [2, 14, 15], in practice it is usually done as a terminal procedure in situ or in isolated lungs [3]. The procedure itself is straightforward and involves administering saline or phosphate-buffered saline into the lungs through the trachea, then withdrawing the fluid. However, care must be taken not to puncture the trachea or lung and to avoid introducing blood into the lungs. In a typical experiment, cells in the BAL fluid are assessed for red blood cell (RBC) count and total leukocyte numbers, with a particular focus on the increased presence of neutrophils as an indicator of inflammation and of RBCs and WBCs with enhanced alveocapillary permeability. The fluid is centrifuged and the cell pellet used for other assays, such as differential staining to assess leukocyte identity and numbers (Section "BAL total cell counts (leukocytes and red blood cells) and differential staining"), or for RNA or protein analysis. The cell-free supernatant can be used to evaluate total protein content (Section "Total protein determination in BAL"), with higher levels relative to baseline taken as additional evidence of increased permeability. Levels of cytokines and other soluble mediators can also be measured. Other procedures that harness the utility of the BAL technique can be employed to further assess permeability, as described in Section "Incorporation of fluorescent dextran into the BAL technique." The literature shows that laboratories often differ in the specifics of how BAL is performed, particularly in volume of saline used, the number of lavages done on a single specimen, and the subsequent processing of the BAL fluid. In most protocols, EDTA (from 0.6 mM up to 10 mM) is added to the saline or PBS to enhance the recovery of attached leukocytes (particularly macrophages). If multiple lavages are done, typically only the first one is used for determining protein concentration, as there is progressive dilution of the protein with continued lavage. All subsequent lavages are pooled to assess the cells. We describe below the procedures we use in our laboratory for the collection, processing, and analysis of BAL fluid and its components.

Basic Technique for in Situ BAL of Euthanized Mice

Materials:

- Isoflurane or euthanasia solution (390 mg/ml pentobarbital sodium and 50 mg/ml phenytoin sodium)
- Sterile Ca^{2+}- and Mg^{2+}-free PBS containing 0.6 mM EDTA, prewarmed to 37 °C
- 1-cc sterile syringe
- Scissors and curved forceps
- 3–0 (USP) silk surgical suture, cut into 12- to 15-cm lengths
- 20-G × 0.5 in. tubing adapter (BD Medical, catalog #408210) or blunt needle (Brico Medical Supplies, catalog #BN2005), sterile (Fig. 4.1a)
- 1.5-ml polypropylene microcentrifuge tubes.

General Procedure:

1. Euthanize the mouse either by exposure to 100 % isoflurane or intraperitoneal injection of a commercially available euthanasia solution.
2. Place the mouse on a Styrofoam support in a flat supine position, with its head facing the investigator, and pin each foreleg.
3. Spray the abdomen with 70 % ethanol. Starting at the xiphoid process cut the skin and membrane over the peritoneal cavity. Push aside the intestines and cut the inferior vena cava (IVC) next to the right kidney (Fig. 4.1b) to bleed out the animal.[1] Use a piece of gauze to capture the blood.
4. Tape down the snout to straighten out the airway and spray the area from the chin to the diaphragm with 70 % ethanol.
5. Starting at the chin of the mouse, cut the skin over the trachea and chest down to the diaphragm. Using forceps pull the salivary glands apart to expose the trachea and surrounding musculature (Fig. 4.1c). Carefully tease away the muscle tissue so that the cartilage rings of the trachea are evident (Fig. 4.1d).
6. Cut along the center of the ribcage to just above the diaphragm, keeping the scissors flush against the sternum to avoid puncturing the underlying heart or lungs, then cut along both sides of the ribcage. Using forceps, carefully pull apart the ribcage at the top and pin down on each side (Fig. 4.1e).

---

[1]This step can be omitted if blood is to be collected.

7. Gently position curved forceps under the trachea and use the forceps to pull a segment of suture underneath the trachea from one side to the other. Loosely tie the suture around the trachea close to the top of the ribcage[2] (Fig. 4.1f).

8. Using the tips of sharp scissors, make a nick in the trachea as close to the pharynx as possible (Fig. 4.1f). Insert a 20-G tubing adapter or blunt needle into the trachea and move it forward. Tighten the suture around the trachea and make another knot (Fig. 4.1g).

9. Attach a 1-cc syringe containing 1 ml[3] of warm PBS/EDTA to the tubing adapter or blunt needle. Slowly push in the entire volume, making sure that all lobes inflate (Fig. 4.1h). Then carefully pull back on the plunger to withdraw as much fluid as possible.[4] If the pressure is high and fluid stops entering the syringe, try carefully adjusting the position of the adapter/needle. Alternatively, the syringe may need to be removed, and a Pipetman fitted with a tip can be used to collect the remaining fluid from the adapter/needle.

10. Transfer the lavage fluid[5] to a microcentrifuge tube, noting the volume recovered, and place on ice.[6]

Incorporation of Fluorescent Dextran into the BAL Technique

To assess permeability changes that accompany ALI, investigators have tradition-ally relied on using albumin or high molecular weight dextrans as tracers. Some approaches involve intranasal or tracheal administration of the tracer to measure its passage into the plasma [1]. Alternatively, the tracer can be added to a lung per-fusate ex vivo or injected in vivo to monitor its accumulation in extravascular compartments. When using albumin as the tracer, it can be radioactively or fluorescently labeled and introduced into the animal, or the endogenous protein can be measured in BAL by colorimetric assays, ELISA, or binding of Evans Blue dye. Our group prefers to use a fluorescent dextran, such as fluorescein isothiocyanate (FITC)-dextran, because it is extremely stable at physiological pH and temperature with little risk of loss of the fluorescent label [4], and analysis requires minimal processing. Using a fluorescent compound also avoids the issue of dealing with radioactive waste. FITC-dextran is intravenously injected into the animal several hours prior to the lavage. Both blood and BAL are then collected, with the aim of

---

[2]If the left lobe is not to be lavaged (for example, if it is intended for an assay in which prior manipulation is contraindicated), it can be tied off at the bronchus using a separate suture. Carefully tease away the pleura attaching the left lobe to the cavity, lift up the lobe using the curved forceps, and slide the suture underneath.

[3]If the left lobe is tied off, we use a volume of 0.8 ml to lavage the right lung.

[4]A typical recovery is 75–90 % of the fluid volume.

[5]Injured mice often yield a BAL that is visibly bloody.

[6]If the left lobe is tied off, at this point it can be removed by cutting below the suture. We usually weigh the lobe and flash freeze it for downstream applications.

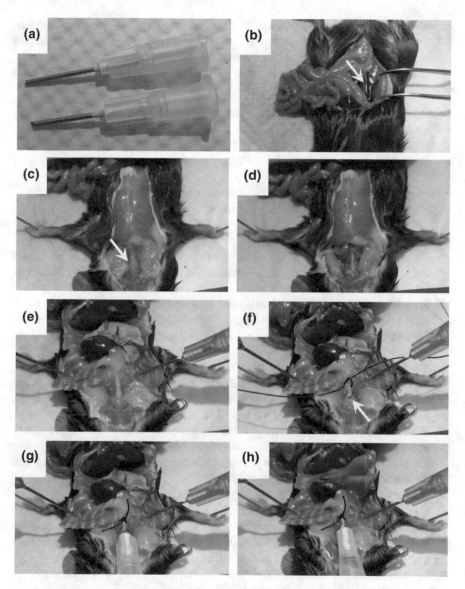

Fig. 4.1 Preparation of the mouse for BAL fluid collection and inflation of the lungs in situ with saline/PBS. **a** Twenty-gauge blunt needle (*top*) and beveled tubing adapter (*bottom*) for insertion into the trachea. **b** The *arrow* indicates the abdominal inferior vena cava. **c** The *arrow* points to the exposed trachea, flanked by the salivary glands and still covered by the musculature. **d** Dissection of the musculature reveals the cartilage rings of the trachea. **e** The thoracic cavity is shown completely open and the ribcage pinned on each side. This mouse was not injured, so the lung lobes appear healthy and pink. **f** A small nick (*arrow*) has been made in the trachea near the pharynx. The suture is loosely tied around the trachea at this step. **g** The adapter is inserted into the trachea through the nick and held in place by knotting the suture twice. **h** Inflation of the lung lobes is clearly evident after introduction of 1 ml PBS/EDTA using a 1-cc syringe attached to the adapter

measuring the concentration of fluorescent dextran in the BAL, normalized to that in the plasma. In this assay, increased fluorescent dextran in the airspace would be a significant indicator of enhanced vascular and epithelial permeability.

Materials (in addition to those listed in Section "Basic technique for in situ BAL of euthanized mice"):

- 70 kDa FITC-dextran, dissolved in sterile PBS to 10 μM (or 0.7 mg/ml)
- Sterile 1-cc syringe and 26-G needle
- Greiner MiniCollect tube containing EDTA (catalog #450474)
- Sterile 3-cc syringe and 25-G needle
- 0.1 M EDTA, pH 7–8
- 96-well assay plate, black with clear bottom
- Microplate reader with fluorescence measurement capability.

General Procedure:

1. Three hours prior to lavage, anesthetize the mouse by exposure to isoflurane and, using the 1-cc syringe and 26-G needle, intravenously[7] inject 100 μl of 10 μM FITC-dextran.
2. Euthanize the mouse by intraperitoneal injection of a commercially available euthanasia solution and expose the thoracic cavity as described in Section "Basic technique for in situ BAL of euthanized mice," omitting the IVC cut.
3. Draw up a ml or so of 0.1 M EDTA into the 3-cc syringe and 25-G needle and expel (this coats the interior of the needle and syringe with anticoagulant without adding substantial volume). With the bevel side of the needle facing up, puncture the right ventricle of the heart and slowly draw blood into the syringe. Withdraw the needle and syringe from the heart.
4. Pull back on the plunger slightly, remove the needle and insert the syringe into the MiniCollect tube. Press the plunger to transfer blood from the syringe into the tube.
5. Gently mix the contents and place the tube on ice.
6. Harvest BAL fluid as described in Section "Basic technique for in situ BAL of euthanized mice."
7. Centrifuge the BAL fluid at 4700–5200 × g for 5 min. Remove the supernatant and place on ice.[8] Proceed with cell pellet as desired for other analyses.
8. Centrifuge the blood at 4700–5200 × g for 10 min at 4 °C. Remove the supernatant (plasma) and transfer to a fresh tube.[9]
9. Prepare dilutions of plasma and BAL (typically in the range of 1:5 for BAL and 1:20 or 1:50 for plasma) and FITC-dextran for the standard curve (ranging from 0.05 to 50 nM).

---

[7]Either via the retro-orbital sinus or tail vein.

[8]Keep BAL and plasma protected from light.

[9]Both BAL and plasma can be stored up to 48 h at −20 °C before the fluorescence measurement.

10. Pipet 100 μl of each dilution, in duplicate or triplicate, into each well of the assay plate.

11. Measure fluorescence using the microplate reader at an excitation wavelength of 493 nm and emission wavelength of 517 nm.

12. Average the fluorescence readings for the standards and plot them as a function of FITC-dextran concentration. Determine the y-intercept and slope using a best-fit line.

13. Average the fluorescence values for the BAL and plasma. Calculate the FITC-dextran concentration using the y-intercept and slope derived from the standard curve in #12 [using equation ((Average OD_{595} − y-intercept) ÷ slope) × dilution factor].[10]

14. Express values as a ratio of fluorescence in the BAL relative to the plasma.[11]

BAL Total Cell Counts (Leukocytes and Red Blood Cells) and Differential Staining

BAL fluid is usually leveraged to obtain a qualitative and quantitative picture of the degree of inflammation and enhanced permeability, both hallmarks of ALI. Total numbers of cells can be assessed by manually counting a small sample of the BAL (either neat or diluted), typically using a hemacytometer. In addition, the composition of the leukocytes is evaluated by morphology coupled with differential staining, a process that employs more than one chemical dye to help the investigator differentiate the cell types from one another. The staining technique was developed by Dmitri Romanowsky and further modified by others (Wright, Giemsa, Leishman) [5, 6, 17–19] to combine methanol-based fixation and staining in a single step, using the basic dye methylene blue to detect nucleic acid and the acidic dye eosin to detect protein. Commercial kits (variously known as Diff-Quik, Diff-Quick, or Kwik-Diff™) are readily available that split the fixation and staining into three separate steps. A sample of cells from the BAL is smeared or centrifuged onto glass slides and taken through the staining process, which is extremely rapid and easy to perform. As previously mentioned, in ALI the expectation is that the total number of leukocytes will be elevated, with increased permeability and transmigration from the tissue through the epithelium into the airspace. The presence and load of neutrophils, which are rarely seen in the airspace at baseline, are particularly indicative of early stages of injury.

---

[10]In BAL from rodents at baseline, we and others have observed the FITC-dextran concentration to be <1 nM, using an administered dose of 10 μM. This level in the BAL fluid can increase by an order of magnitude with injury.

[11]The concentration of FITC-dextran can also be expressed as mg FITC-dextran per ml BAL fluid and compared to levels in uninjured mice.

Materials:

- Lavage fluid from Section "Basic technique for in situ BAL of euthanized mice"
- 1X and 10X PBS
- Bright-Line™ hemacytometer, Improved Neubauer (Hausser Scientific), with glass coverslip
- Crystal violet, 0.01 % (in 1 % (v/v) glacial acetic acid)
- Inverted phase microscope
- 0.5- and 1.5-ml polypropylene microcentrifuge tubes
- Microcentrifuge
- Shandon Cytoslide (Thermo Scientific, catalog #5991056)
- EZ Single Cytofunnel (Thermo Scientific, catalog #5991040)
- Shandon Cytospin 3 instrument (or equivalent)
- Shandon Kwik-Diff™ Staining kit (Thermo Scientific, catalog #9990700)
- Coplin jars or 50-ml conical polypropylene tubes for staining
- Conventional microscope with bright field capability.

General Procedure:

1. Clean the hemacytometer and cover glass with 70 % ethanol and dry each with a Kimwipe. Place the coverslip over the central chamber of the hemacytometer.
2. Carefully pipet 10 µl of the BAL fluid under the coverslip and allow the cells to settle. At the microscope, use the 40× objective to count the number of red blood cells (RBCs) in 4 corner 1-mm^2 squares of the hemacytometer (each of these corner squares is further divided into 16 smaller squares)[12,13] One of the 4 corner squares is highlighted in yellow in Fig. 4.2a. Add these 4 values and multiply the sum by 2500 to obtain the number of RBCs per ml.[14] For BAL that is overtly bloody, count the RBCs in 5 diagonal squares (highlighted in blue in Fig. 4.2a) out of the 25 that comprise the central area of the chamber. Add these 5 values and multiply the sum by 50,000 to obtain the number of RBCs per ml.[15]
3. Using the 20× objective, count the white blood cells (WBCs) in the 4 corner squares.[16] Calculate the cell concentration as described in item #2.[17] Figure 4.2b shows the size differential between leukocytes and RBCs.

---

[12]Each corner square is surrounded by triple lines. Cells within the triple lines are counted, as well as cells that touch the lines on two perpendicular sides (but not on the other two sides) (Fig. 4.2a).

[13]Ideally, a total of 100–200 cells should be counted for the most accurate determination.

[14]The RBC concentration range in BAL fluid from uninjured mice (using 1 ml saline for the lavage) is typically 10^4–10^5 cells per ml.

[15]Alternatively, BAL can be diluted for counting RBCs in the 4 corner squares. Any dilution amount needs to be factored into the calculation to obtain cells per ml.

[16]If desired, crystal violet can be used to visualize WBCs: Mix 20 µl BAL with 20 µl crystal violet and count WBCs in the 4 corner 1-mm^2 squares of the hemacytometer. Add values and multiply by 2500 *and* by 2 to obtain WBCs per ml.

[17]The leukocyte count in BAL fluid (1 ml used for lavage) from animals at baseline usually ranges from 1 to 2 × 10^5 cells/ml.

Fig. 4.2 Counting cells with a hemacytometer. **a** The grid layout of an Improved Neubauer hemacytometer is illustrated. One of the 4 corner squares, composed of 16 smaller squares, is highlighted in *yellow*. By convention, cells (*gray circles*) within or touching the lines defining the perimeter of the yellow square are counted, excluding cells on the *top* and *right* side, as shown by the X's. The internal squares highlighted in *blue* are used for counting red blood cells (RBCs) when they are numerous in the BAL fluid. **b** Photomicrograph at 400× depicting cells in 10 µl BAL fluid (harvested from an uninjured mouse) loaded into a hemacytometer. The arrows point to leukocytes and the arrowhead indicates an RBC (note the size difference)

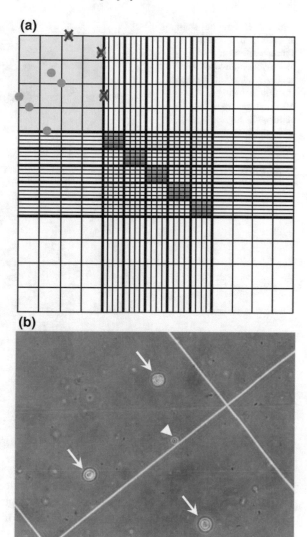

4. Centrifuge the BAL fluid at 4700–5200 × *g* for 5 min.
5. Remove the supernatant and save at −20 °C for later protein analysis (see Section "Total protein determination in BAL").
6. Resuspend the cell pellet in H_2O,[18] rapidly (within 30 s) followed by the appropriate volume of 10X PBS, to yield a concentration of ~1.5 × 10^5 cells/ml.

---

[18]This step results in lysis of the RBCs.

Fig. 4.3 Differential staining
of cells in BAL fluid
harvested from a
bleomycin-injured mouse
at day 7. Photomicrographs
at 400× showing
macrophages (*arrows*),
neutrophils (*arrowheads*),
and lymphocytes (*asterisks*)
after cytospinning cells from
BAL and staining with
Kwik-Diff™

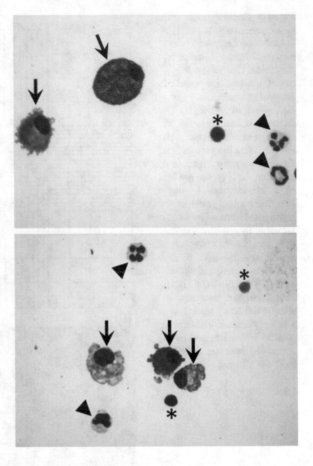

7. Load a cytoslide into a cytofunnel and snap it closed. Pipet 200 μl, or ~30,000 cells, into the chamber of the cytofunnel. Centrifuge in a Cytospin 3 for 2 min at 1000 rpm (use a balance cytofunnel and slide if only one sample is being centrifuged). After removing the cytofunnel from the centrifuge, carefully open and remove the slide. Allow the slide to air dry.

8. Stain the slide sequentially in Kwik-Diff ™ solutions 1 through 3 by dipping 5 times in each solution, 1 s each. Between each solution, drain any excess into the container and blot the edge of the slide on a paper towel. Once staining is complete, rinse the slide in distilled H_2O and let it air dry vertically.

9. Under the microscope and using the 20× objective, count at least 300 cells total (we typically count 450), tallying the number of neutrophils (clear cytoplasm with blue segmented nuclear material), macrophages (large cells with blue nucleus and prominent, often granular blue cytoplasm), and lymphocytes (small cells with blue nucleus and little cytoplasm) (Fig. 4.3). Eosinophils (blue

segmented nucleus and distinctive pink granules in the cytoplasm)[19] may occasionally be observed, but these cells are more typical in allergic inflammation rather than acute injury. It is recommended to report both the percentage and total number of each leukocyte type.

Total Protein Determination in BAL

A colorimetric assay to measure total protein content in the BAL fluid is a technically simple way to assess protein leak in lung injury. The most typical assay used is based on the Bradford method, in which binding of the Coomassie blue dye to protein at an acidic pH causes the absorption maximum to shift from 465 to 595 nm (along with a change in color of the dye from brown to blue). One caveat to keep in mind is that the protein level in BAL can also be impacted by high filtration pressures and altered cardiac output, in addition to enhanced permeability [13]. Total protein measurements can be coupled with analysis of a specific tracer, such as described above in C, to enhance confidence in concluding that permeability is increased in the ALI model being investigated.

Materials:

- Cell-free lavage fluid from Section "BAL total cell counts (leukocytes and red blood cells) and differential staining"
- Bradford protein assay reagent (our group has used kits from Bio-Rad and Pierce (catalog #23200), both of which include the protein binding dye and bovine serum albumin (BSA) as a standard. In the Bio-Rad kit, the dye reagent (catalog #500-0006) is provided as a concentrate that requires dilution, and bovine gamma globulin (catalog #500-0001) is available as an alternative standard to BSA. The protocol below is for the Bio-Rad kit)
- 96-well assay plate
- Microplate mixer (optional)
- Microplate reader
- Whatman #1 filter paper and funnel for preparation of dye reagent.

General Procedure:

1. Dilute 1 part dye reagent concentrate with 4 parts distilled H_2O. Filter through Whatman paper folded to fit in a glass funnel. Diluted reagent can be stored for 2 weeks at room temperature.
2. Reconstitute standard (we typically use BSA) according to the manufacturer's protocol. Prepare four to five dilutions of the BSA standard, ranging from 0.05 to 0.5 mg/ml (linear range of the assay).

---

[19]Alveolar macrophages are the dominant cell type in BAL from uninjured mice. Basophils are rarely observed in BAL fluid.

3. Dilute BAL from injured mice from 1:5 to 1:20 (BAL from naïve mice is assayed neat).
4. Pipet 10 μl of each standard dilution and each BAL sample into wells (two or three wells per standard/sample).
5. Add 200 μl of diluted dye reagent to each well. Mix by pipetting up and down or shake the plate for one minute on a microplate mixer.
6. Incubate 5 min at room temperature, then measure the absorbance at 595 nm within one hour[20] on a microplate reader.
7. Average the OD_{595} values[21] for the standards and plot them as a function of protein concentration. Determine the y-intercept and slope using a best-fit line.[22]
8. Average the OD_{595} values for the BAL unknowns. Calculate the BAL protein concentration in mg/ml[23] using the y-intercept and slope derived from the standard curve in #7 [using equation ((Average OD_{595} − y-intercept) ÷ slope) × dilution factor (if required)].

Lung Tissue Processing and Analysis

As mentioned in the introduction to this chapter, evaluation of the lungs by histology and light microscopy provides another vital measure of the extent of injury in mouse models of ALI. In a typical experiment, lungs are collected after cannulating the trachea, inflated with a formaldehyde-based fixative, embedded in paraffin, sectioned, and stained with hematoxylin (nucleus) and eosin (protein). Features that are looked for include neutrophil infiltration into the alveolar space, walls, and interstitium, alveolar wall and interstitial thickening, hemorrhage, alveolar congestion with proteinaceous debris and fibrin deposition (known as hyaline membranes), and alveolar and perivascular edema. Whether all or only some of these features are observed often depends on the type of injury. As part of the injury repair process, collagen is synthesized and deposited in the lung interstitium, where it can be quantified histologically (by picrosirius red staining and morphometric analysis) or by several biochemical assays. The Sircol™ collagen assay is a dye-based method that measures acid-soluble fragments of pepsin-digested collagen. Another assay assesses the content of hydroxyproline, which results from hydroxylation of proline and is almost exclusive to collagen. In this

---

[20] Absorbance values will increase over time.

[21] The coefficient of variance (CV), which is the standard deviation divided by the average and multiplied by 100, ideally should be <10 % for replicates.

[22] Alternatively, microplate reader software can be used to calculate the concentration of unknowns based on the standards, and a four-parameter (quadratic) fit generally gives more reliable data than a linear fit.

[23] Total protein in BAL from uninjured mice normally ranges from 100 to 200 μg/ml, whereas in our experience the level increases at least an order of magnitude with acute injury.

section, we present our technique for ensuring adequate inflation of mouse lungs prior to fixation for histological staining. In addition, we briefly discuss a simple scoring regimen advocated by the ATS Workshop [8] for quantitative assessment of injury in lung sections from animal models of ALI. Finally, we provide the method we most commonly use to measure collagen levels in injured mouse lungs.

Lung Inflation and Fixation

Proper inflation of the lung is critically important for reliable interpretation of changes in morphological features. A pressure range of 15–25 cm H_2O is generally recommended, as this allows fixation at functional residual capacity (volume of air in the lungs after passive expiration) [8]. Below we describe our setup and procedure for dissection and inflation of mouse lungs. Note that if inflation and fixation of the lungs are done after the lavage has been performed, sections from such tissue will not be representative of the inflammatory cell content in the airspaces.

Materials:

- Formaldehyde-based fixative[24]
- 60-cc syringe, with plunger removed
- Tubing with stopcock
- Scissors and two pairs of curved forceps
- Vascular clamp (Schwartz Micro Serrefines) with sharp bend (Fine Science Tools, catalog #18052-03)
- 50-ml polypropylene conical tubes.

General Procedure:

1. Affix the syringe to a support (we tape it to a glass graduated cylinder), tip facing down. Attach tubing to the syringe tip. The end of the tubing (with the stopcock) should be immobilized at 15–25 cm from the syringe tip (Fig. 4.4a).
2. Pour 30 ml of fixative into the syringe barrel.
3. After euthanizing the mouse and cannulating the trachea as described in Section "Basic technique for in situ BAL of euthanized mice,"[25] use forceps to grasp the trachea, with the adapter/blunt needle still in place. Carefully cut away the tissue under the trachea using scissors.

---

[24]We generally use 4 % paraformaldehyde, although buffered formalin is an excellent alternative and other fixatives can be substituted as well. If prepared in the lab, paraformaldehyde should be fresh or used within a week (and stored at 4 °C or frozen). We also purchase 16 % paraformaldehyde from Electron Microscopy Sciences (catalog #15710) and dilute that to 4 % with PBS (store at 4 °C).

[25]As described in Section "Basic technique for in situ BAL of euthanized mice," the left lung (or the right lung) can be tied off at the bronchus with a separate suture, if desired for other assays.

Fig. 4.4 Inflation of lungs
with fixative. **a** The setup in
our laboratory for inflation
and fixation of harvested
lungs, which are shown
before (**b**) and after
(**c**) inflation with 4 %
paraformaldehyde. The
distance between the fixative
and the lungs is indicated
(yielding a pressure of 20 cm
H_2O)

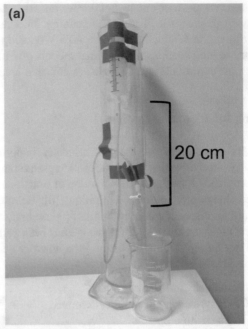

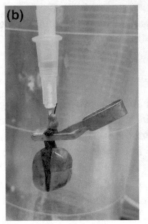
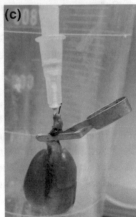

4. Still holding the trachea with one pair of forceps, use the other pair to tease and
   pull away tissue from the underside of the lungs, taking care not to tear the lung
   tissue.
5. Use scissors to cut the IVC and release the lungs, heart, and thymus from the
   thoracic cavity en bloc.
6. Place the vascular clamp on the trachea to keep it attached to the adapter/blunt
   needle. Affix the adapter/blunt needle to the stopcock of the tubing.

7. Open the stopcock and allow fixative to flow through the lungs for about 10 min, using a flow rate of 1 drop per second. Lobes should fully inflate (Fig. 4.4b, c).
8. Close the stopcock, remove the adapter/blunt needle from the stopcock, and remove the vascular clamp to release the tissue.
9. Immerse the lungs in 20–25 ml of fixative for 24 h at 4 °C, with gentle rocking.[26]
10. Rinse tissue with PBS and store in 70 % ethanol at 4 °C until ready to embed.[27]

Assessment of Injury in Lung Tissue Sections

Sections of lungs that were inflated as described in Section "Lung inflation and fixation" are typically stained with hematoxylin and eosin and examined by light microscopy for a qualitative and quantitative assessment of injury. As mentioned in the introductory comments to this section, injury is accompanied by one or more characteristic features, depending on the nature of the injury. Matute-Bello et al. recently developed an elegantly simple scoring system to facilitate quantification of injury [8]. In this system, each of 5 variables is assigned a weighted value; these variables include, in descending order of relevance, (1) neutrophils in the alveolar space, (2) neutrophils in the interstitial space and alveolar walls, (3) presence of hyaline membranes, (4) presence of proteinaceous deposits in the alveolar air-spaces, and (5) thickening of the alveolar septa to at least twice the normal size. Using this scoring system requires that investigators become familiar with the specific features manifested in their injury model. For example, the ATS Workshop on ALI notes that hyaline membranes, seen as solid bands of eosin-stained material and characteristic of ALI in human, are rarely observed in lungs of mice [8]. This is a variable that an investigator could elect to omit if the model warrants. In our own studies examining early time points in the bleomycin injury model, we are most interested in the quantity and localization of neutrophils and thickening of the alveolar walls (Fig. 4.5). Regardless which features are chosen for scoring, it is critical to define those variables and how scoring is performed, to assess sections in a blinded fashion, to select microscopic fields randomly, and to evaluate enough fields (at least 20, observed at 400×, are recommended by the ATS Workshop on ALI) to be representative of the injury as a whole.

---

[26]For frozen sections, we generally fix the lungs for 2 h at room temperature and transfer to cold 18–30 % sucrose overnight. Lungs are then immersed in Optimal Cutting Temperature (OCT) compound added to an appropriately sized cryomold and frozen in a dry ice/ethanol bath.
[27]If desired, cut away the heart and thymus before embedding the lungs in paraffin or OCT.

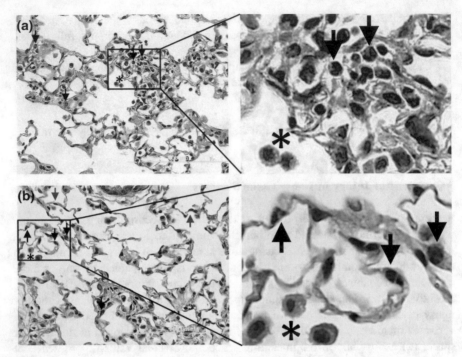

Fig. 4.5 Histological evidence of acute lung injury. Shown are photomicrographs (400×, *yellow lines* in panels **a** and **b** denote 100 μm) of sections, stained with hematoxylin and eosin, from the lungs of 2 mice injured with bleomycin 7 days before harvest. The *boxed* regions in each panel are also displayed at an additional 4× magnification to the right. The *black arrows* point to neutrophils in the interstitium and alveolar walls and *asterisks* indicate macrophages in the alveolar space. Because the lungs were lavaged before harvest in this experiment, neutrophils, usually less abundant than macrophages, are essentially absent from the alveolar space. The alveolar walls and interstitium show significant thickening, although in panel **b**, areas with thin, normally appearing alveolar walls are evident (*red arrows*)

Biochemical Analysis of Collagen

To quantitatively assess collagen in the lungs, our laboratory has traditionally favored the hydroxyproline assay, originally developed 65 years ago [11] and further modified by many other investigators since then. In this assay, acid hydrolysates of lung tissue are subjected to oxidation by chloramine T and then reacted with dimethylaminobenzaldehyde, forming a dark red product in proportion to the level of hydroxyproline (and thus collagen). We usually perform this assay using the left lung as it is easy to isolate from the right lung lobes. The following two-day protocol incorporates laboratory-made reagents, although commercial kits are also available (for example, see Sigma catalog #MAK008).

Materials:

- Hydroxyproline standard (Sigma, catalog# H-1637)
- Chloramine solution, prepared fresh (0.7 g chloramines T (Sigma, catalog #C-9887), 45 ml 0.5 M sodium acetate, pH 6.0, 5 ml of isopropanol)
- Erlich's solution (14.9 g *p*-dimethylaminobenzaldehyde (Sigma, catalog #D8904), 70 ml isopropanol, 20 ml of 100 % perchloric acid, and 10 ml H_2O. Store at 4 °C protected from light for up to 1 month).
- 6 N, 1 N, and 0.001 N HCl
- 6 N and 1 N NaOH
- Clear glass threaded vials with caps (Fisher, catalog #14-955-325)
- Scissors and razor blades
- Petri dish
- Spatula
- Oven capable of 110 °C
- 5-cc syringes and 18-G needles
- 15-ml conical polypropylene tubes
- syringe filters, 0.45 μm
- pH meter and electrode OR pH paper/strips
- water bath set to 65 °C
- 96-well assay plate
- Microplate reader.

General Procedure[28]:

1. Prepare hydroxyproline at 100 mg/ml in 0.001 N HCl (store at 4 °C protected from light). Make a twofold dilution series from 200 to 3.125 μg/ml (fresh for each experiment).
2. Thaw the lung specimen from the freezer and finely mince it using sharp tipped scissors and a razor blade in a petri dish.
3. Use a spatula to collect the minced tissue and transfer it into a glass vial containing 1 ml 6 N HCl. Ensure all pieces of tissue are immersed in HCl and tightly cap the vial.[29]
4. Incubate the sample in an oven at 110 °C overnight.
5. Next day, remove the vial from the oven and let it cool to room temperature. Add 1 ml 6 N NaOH.
6. Draw up the sample into a 5-cc syringe, using an 18-G needle. Pass the sample through a 0.45-μm syringe filter into a 15-ml tube.

---

[28]Our protocol was originally provided by Dr. Carol Feghali-Bostwick's laboratory.

[29]The kit from Sigma uses a smaller amount of tissue and volume than called for in our protocol. In addition, after hydrolysis, a portion of the sample (5–25 %) is added to the 96-well plate and either dried under vacuum or in an oven at 60 °C. This step obviates the need to adjust the pH.

7. Add 4 ml distilled H_2O to the sample and adjust the pH of the sample to between 6 and 9 using 1 N HCl and 1 N NaOH. Check using pH meter.[30]
8. Record the new volume of the sample.
9. Add 100 µl of the sample and each standard individually to 1 ml chloramine solution and incubate at room temperature for 20 min. The samples will usually appear pale yellow whereas the standards remain colorless.
10. Add 1 ml of Erlich's solution to each sample and standard and incubate at 65 °C for 15 min.
11. Transfer 200 µl of each reaction mixture, in triplicate, to a 96-well plate.
12. Measure absorbance at 570 nm using a microplate reader.
13. Average the OD_{570} values for the standards and plot them as a function of hydroxyproline concentration. Determine the y-intercept and slope using a best-fit line.
14. Average the triplicate OD_{570} values for the lung sample. Calculate the hydroxyproline concentration in µg/ml using the y-intercept and slope derived from the standard curve in #13 (using equation (Average OD_{595} − y-intercept) ÷ slope).
15. Multiply the µg/ml value by the sample volume in #8 to obtain µg of hydroxyproline per left lung.[31]

Acknowledgments The authors thank previous members of Lynn Schnapp's laboratory for their practical contributions to these protocols. We also thank Dr. Sarah Stephenson for reading the manuscript and Dr. Tetsuya Nishimoto for help with details of the hydroxyproline assay.

References

1. Chen H, Wu S, Lu R, Zhang YG, Zheng Y, Sun J. Pulmonary permeability assessed by fluorescent-labeled dextran instilled intranasally into mice with lps-induced acute lung injury. PLoS ONE. 2014;9(7):e101925.
2. Dames C, Akyuz L, Reppe K, Tabeling C, Dietert K, Kershaw O, et al. Miniaturized bronchoscopy enables unilateral investigation, application, and sampling in mice. Am J Respir Cell Mol Biol. 2014;51(6):730–7.
3. Daubeuf F, Frossard N. Performing bronchoalveolar lavage in the mouse. Curr Protoc Mouse Biol. 2012;2(2):167–75.
4. Guery BP, Nelson S, Viget N, Fialdes P, Summer WR, Dobard E, et al. Fluorescein-labeled dextran concentration is increased in bal fluid after antu-induced edema in rats. J Appl Physiol (1985). 1998;85(3):842–8.

---

[30]Alternatively, omit addition of the H_2O and use pH paper/strips to check the pH. Vortex the sample between drops of HCl and NaOH. Adjusting the pH is the most time-consuming step in the procedure, especially if a large number of samples is being analyzed.

[31]In uninjured mice, expect a range of 30–40 µg hydroxyproline per left lung. As a reference, this range typically increases to 60–80 at day 21 post bleomycin (a time point characterized by significant fibrosis during the resolution phase of injury).

5. Horobin RW, Walter KJ. Understanding romanowsky staining. I: the romanowsky-giemsa effect in blood smears. Histochemistry. 1987;86(3):331–6.
6. Leishman WB. Note on a simple and rapid method of producing romanowsky staining in malarial and other blood films. Br Med J. 1901;2(2125):757–8.
7. Martin TR, Matute-Bello G. Experimental models and emerging hypotheses for acute lung injury. Crit Care Clin. 2011;27(3):735–52.
8. Matute-Bello G, Downey G, Moore BB, Groshong SD, Matthay MA, Slutsky AS, et al. An official american thoracic society workshop report: Features and measurements of experimental acute lung injury in animals. Am J Respir Cell Mol Biol. 2011;44(5):725–38.
9. Matute-Bello G, Frevert CW, Martin TR. Animal models of acute lung injury. Am J Physiol Lung Cell Mol Physiol. 2008;295(3):L379–99.
10. Mizgerd JP, Skerrett SJ. Animal models of human pneumonia. Am J Physiol Lung Cell Mol Physiol. 2008;294(3):L387–98.
11. Neuman RE, Logan MA. The determination of hydroxyproline. J Biol Chem. 1950;184 (1):299–306.
12. Parker JC. Acute lung injury and pulmonary vascular permeability: use of transgenic models. Compr Physiol. 2011;1(2):835–82.
13. Parker JC, Townsley MI. Evaluation of lung injury in rats and mice. Am J Physiol Lung Cell Mol Physiol. 2004;286(2):L231–46.
14. Polikepahad S, Barranco WT, Porter P, Anderson B, Kheradmand F, Corry DB. A reversible, non-invasive method for airway resistance measurements and bronchoalveolar lavage fluid sampling in mice. J Vis Exp. 2010;38:1720.
15. Walters DM, Wills-Karp M, Mitzner W. Assessment of cellular profile and lung function with repeated bronchoalveolar lavage in individual mice. Physiol Genomics. 2000;2(1):29–36.
16. Ware LB. Modeling human lung disease in animals. Am J Physiol Lung Cell Mol Physiol. 2008;294(2):L149–50.
17. Wittekind D. On the nature of romanowsky dyes and the romanowsky-giemsa effect. Clin Lab Haematol. 1979;1(4):247–62.
18. Woronzoff-Dashkoff KK. The wright-giemsa stain. Secrets revealed. Clin Lab Med. 2002;22 (1):15–23.
19. Wright JH. A rapid method for the differential staining of blood films and malarial parasites. J Med Res. 1902;7(1):138–44.

Chapter 5
Invasive Measurement of Pulmonary Function in Mice

Xiaozhu Huang and Annette Robichaud

Background

Patients surviving ARDS commonly have pulmonary function abnormalities upon discharge including reduction in diffusing capacity, airflow obstruction, or restriction (20 %) on spirometry and lung volumes [27]. The addition of pulmonary function testing to analysis of mouse models of acute lung injury can add to the translational potential of the findings and provide additional insight into the pathophysiologic processes that underlie human diseases [2, 18, 35]. Our understanding of normal and abnormal pulmonary function has clearly benefited from studies of mice [7, 8, 29]. Pulmonary function tests are important tools to quantify phenotypic characteristics of respiratory disease models [1, 9, 13, 16, 38]. However, the valid assessment of pulmonary function in an animal as small as the mouse presents considerable technical challenges. Currently, there are three general approaches used to assess respiratory mechanics in mice. They are: (1) ex vivo techniques requiring removal of the trachea and lungs from animals; (2) in vivo invasive techniques requiring anesthesia and surgery on animals; (3) in vivo noninvasive techniques requiring no anesthesia or surgery. Invasive monitoring of pulmonary function using parameters such as pulmonary resistance (R_L) or dynamic compliance (C_{dyn}) is the classical method for accurate and specific determination of respiratory mechanics. In this discussion, we will be focusing on the in vivo invasive but not noninvasive techniques for pulmonary function studies due to the increasing concerns about the validity of measurements obtained with in vivo noninvasive approaches [3, 28].

X. Huang (✉)
Department of Medicine, University of California, San Francisco, CA, USA
e-mail: xiaozhu.huang@ucsf.edu

A. Robichaud
SCIREQ Scientific Respiratory Equipment Inc., Montreal, QC, Canada

© Springer International Publishing AG 2017
L.M. Schnapp and C. Feghali-Bostwick (eds.), *Acute Lung Injury and Repair*,
Respiratory Medicine, DOI 10.1007/978-3-319-46527-2_5

In Vivo Invasive Techniques

Although there are several disadvantages associated with using in vivo invasive techniques, such as the need for anesthesia, surgery and mechanical ventilation, the invasive recording of pulmonary resistance (R_L) and dynamic compliance (C_{dyn}) provide precise and specific determinations of respiratory mechanics. Currently, two major in vivo invasive systems are commercially available that can measure pulmonary function in mice. One is the DSI's BUXCO Finepointe RC system (St Paul, MN, USA) and the other one is the *flexiVent* system from SCIREQ Inc. (Montreal, QC, Canada). The FinePointe RC system provides highly integrated hardware/software to collect invasive dynamic resistance, compliance, and elastance data in anesthetized animals. The animal is anesthetized and instrumented to directly measure respiratory flow and airway pressure. From these direct measurements of airflow and pressure, R_L and C_{dyn} are computed [12, 32]. BUXCO also offers a separate forced maneuver system that is specifically designed for animal models of COPD. On the other hand, the *flexiVent* is an integrated experimental platform for mechanical ventilation and pulmonary function measurements [24]. The precision piston of this computer-operated and programmable device is used to control and standardize the experimental conditions under which the measurements are taken (e.g., breathing frequency, tidal volume, lung volume), as well as to deliver predefined input sinusoidal oscillations for respiratory mechanics assessment. During the delivery of the test signal, the system captures airway pressure, flow, and volume signals and calculates highly reproducible parameters describing the mechanical properties of the respiratory system [24, 30, 31]. The system uses the classic single-compartment linear model of the lung and linear regression to estimate total respiratory system resistance, elastance, and compliance. In addition, it can provide a detailed assessment of the pulmonary function. This is done by capturing the mechanical properties of conducting airways and lung tissue (which includes terminal airways and parenchyma) through a broadband frequency forced oscillation and the use of advanced mathematical models, such as the constant phase model [17]. This system can also perform pressure-volume curves, recruitment maneuvers, negative pressure-driven forced expirations, as well as being used to minimize motion artifacts during thoracic imaging.

This report attempts to focus on the *flexiVent* system (http://www.scireq.com/flexivent) for measuring pulmonary function in anesthetized mice with special attention to practical considerations. It also reflects our own practical experience in using the system based on studies involving models of allergic airway disease in mice. Emphasis will be put on analyses or "perturbations" (predefined waveforms) typically associated with the *flexiVent* system and that have been commonly used in the studies of respiratory disease. While these analyses share some common requirements, they also possess some unique application characteristics that will be discussed separately.

Animal Preparation Using the *flexiVent* System

All selected *flexiVent* analyses require instrumentation of the trachea in anesthetized animals. Each institution has its own recommended protocol for small animal anesthesia. Our group uses the combination of Ketamine/Xylazine/Acepromazine (100/10/2 mg/kg, respectively) administered intraperitoneally to achieve adequate depth of anesthesia for at least 30 min. It usually takes 5–10 min for the anesthetic to take effect. The adequacy of anesthesia is assessed by the toe-pinch reflex. If the animal attempts to withdraw its limb, it is a sign of it not being sufficiently anesthetized. An extra dose of anesthetic agents should then be administered. Once adequate anesthesia is confirmed, a tracheostomy is performed and a tubing adaptor, such as 20 gauge plastic catheters from Smiths Medical (Southington, CT; typical resistance of 0.3 $cmH_2O.s/mL$) is used to cannulate the trachea. Mice are then attached to the *flexiVent* rodent ventilator/pulmonary mechanics analyzer and ventilated at a tidal volume of 10 ml/kg, a ventilation frequency of 150 breaths/min and a positive end-expiratory pressure (PEEP) of 3 cmH_2O. To avoid the influence of spontaneous breathing efforts, which can spoil the input signal and lead to rejected datasets, mice need to be paralyzed with pancuronium (0.1 mg/kg intraperitoneally). Before executing any measurements, a deep lung inflation maneuver (Deep Inflation or TLC in the early software version) should be performed to open any closed lung areas and to normalize the baseline of each animal.

To assess airway responsiveness, cholinergic bronchoconstrictive agents, such as methacholine/acetylcholine (Mch/Ach) are administered to the animal at increasing doses either by aerosol inhalation or systemically by intravenous administration via the tail or jugular vein. Since different strains of mice respond quite differently to a given bronchoconstrictor agent and may require different doses to produce a similar effect, it is very important for investigators to titrate the dosage so that the optimal response can be achieved.

Airway responsiveness can be assessed by reporting the absolute peak values of the responses, the percentage change from baseline or the area under the curve of the response over time. Each dataset is associated with a coefficient of determination (COD), which is a quality control parameter measuring the goodness of the model fit to the experimental data. Before exporting parameters for analyses, investigators need to pay attention to that coefficient and include only datasets having met the acceptance criteria.

Single Frequency Forced Oscillation

The single frequency forced oscillation (SFFO) uses a 2.5 Hz sinusoidal forcing function (e.g., SnapShot-150) and produces the classical and widely used dynamic resistance and compliance parameters. Three parameters are derived from this analysis which captures the mechanical properties of the whole respiratory system (airways, lungs, and chest wall). These include: (1) Resistance (R_{rs}): this parameter describes the dynamic resistance and quantitatively assesses the overall level of opposition to flow within the respiratory system. (2) Elastance (E_{rs}): this parameter is the dynamic elastance which captures the elastic rigidity or the stiffness of the respiratory system. (3) Compliance (C_{rs}): this parameter is the dynamic compliance. It is the reciprocal of E_{rs} and therefore captures the ease with which the respiratory system can be inflated. SFFO is extremely brief in duration (1.2 s) and can therefore be executed in a closely spaced manner for an enhanced resolution of quick responses over time.

To determine airway responsiveness using this analysis, our group prefers to intravenously administer threefold increasing concentrations of the bronchoconstrictor Ach through an indwelling tail vein catheter. Briefly, a 27 G needle connected to PE10 Polyethylene tubing is placed in the tail vein of the anesthetized and tracheostomized mice and measurements of respiratory mechanics are made continuously using SnapShot-150 perturbation. Mice are given increasing doses of Ach to generate a dose response curve. Our group prefers to work with intravenous administrations of Ach as this enables us to achieve quick responses while minimizing the cumulative effects of multiple doses as this agent is rapidly metabolized. Shown in Fig. 5.1a is the data acquired from multiple mice. This original dataset can be reviewed in the software and exported in a spreadsheet for further analysis. Figure 5.1b demonstrates the extracted peak response in Balb-C and C57BL/6 mice

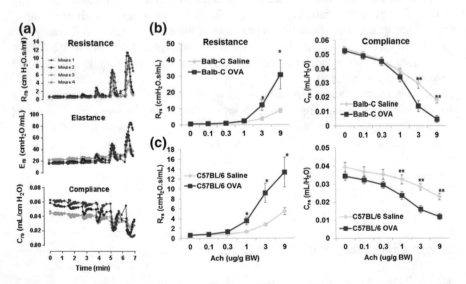

Fig. 5.1 Changes in resistance, elastance and compliance following increasing doses of acetylcholine (Ach) administered intravenously in mice. **a** Example of the response acquired over time in a few mice using a 2.5 Hz single frequency forced oscillation (SnapShot-150). **b, c** Peak resistance and compliance in control and ovalbumin (OVA)-sensitized and challenged Balb-C (**b**) and C57BL/6 (**c**) mice. *$p < 0.05$, **$p < 0.01$

at baseline and after antigen sensitization/challenge. As it is shown, both Balb-C and C57BL/6 mice had significantly increased responsiveness to Ach (measured by either R_{rs} or C_{rs}) after antigen sensitization and challenge compared to unsensitized control mice. In addition, the response of the respiratory system was much more pronounced in the Balb-C than in the C57BL/6 mice, a point which is worth bearing in mind when designing experiments. Based on these results, it is clear that investigators should avoid using mice from mixed genetic backgrounds in similar studies, even if littermates are used as control, since genetic background can introduce large degrees of variability.

Broadband Forced Oscillation

Broadband low-frequency forced oscillations (BBFO) provide an exhaustive assessment of the respiratory system over an extended range of frequencies (1–20.5 Hz) and that in a single perturbation (e.g., Quick Prime-3). As an outcome, this analysis first generates impedance spectra, which are then physiologically interpreted using the constant phase model [17]. This more advanced mathematical model distinguishes between central airway and peripheral tissue mechanics, thus allowing a detailed phenotype characterization of lung diseases in mice. The parameters associated with this analysis include: (1) Newtonian resistance (R_N): this parameter represents the resistance of the central or conducting airways. (2) Tissue damping (G): this parameter closely relates to tissue resistance and reflects the energy dissipation in the lung tissue. (3) Tissue elastance (H): this parameter closely relates to tissue elastance and reflects the energy conservation in the lung tissue. These parameters can provide valuable detailed information and could prove helpful to dissect underlying mechanisms. BBFO can be incorporated in an automated measurement sequence that can include other perturbations for a more comprehensive functional assessment of the respiratory system.

In the example shown in Fig. 5.2, mice were given increasing concentrations of Mch administered as an aerosol through an in-line nebulizer to generate a concentration response curve. This figure illustrates the response over time acquired from multiple mice using this approach. The raw R_N, G, and H values are calculated directly from the software and can later be exported for analysis. Investigators have reported changes of the R_N, G, and H parameters of the constant phase model in studies of lung disease models [23, 24, 26, 36] including allergen-induced pulmonary physiology changes [6, 19, 34]. Despite that, our group, which has been using the *flexiVent* system for studies of allergic lung inflammation for many years, has been focusing on the SSFO described above to assess AHR in these models primarily because the protocol used in our laboratory (i.e., increasing doses of Ach administered intravenously) induces a quick response and high levels of bronchoconstriction. Since the constant phase model is best suited for moderate levels of bronchoconstriction, this often leads in our experimental conditions to a poor fit of the constant phase model to impedance spectra, especially at higher doses of Ach. As a consequence, we are often faced with the impossibility to use parameters, such

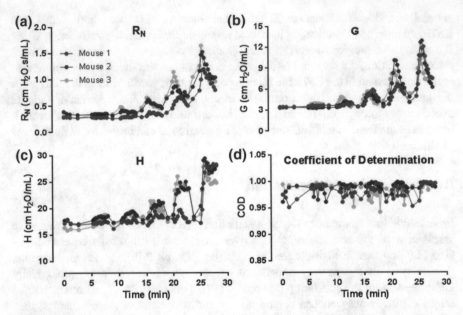

Fig. 5.2 Changes in airway resistance (R_N), tissue damping (G) and tissue elastance (H) following increasing challenges of aerosolized methacholine in mice. **Panel a, b,** and **c** provide an example of the response acquired over time in a few mice using a broadband frequency forced oscillation (Quick Prime-3). In **panel d**, the coefficient of determination describing the fit of the constant phase model to the impedance spectra is reported

as R_N, G, or H to detect AHR because of rejected datasets. However, the impedance spectra remain valid and can always be used to assess AHR at a specific frequency [10] or with other mathematical models describing the mechanical properties of the respiratory system. Alternatively, the situation can be addressed by modifying the dose-range of the bronchoconstrictor agent or by assessing AHR using aerosol deliveries of increasing Mch concentrations, where the exposure would be less. In this latter approach, care must be taken to avoid that condensation accumulates inside the tracheal catheter and obstructs the delivery of the test signal, which would have an important negative effect on the measurement. Carefully cleaning the aerosol delivery line between each subject is, in our view, very helpful in preventing that technical issue.

Quasi-Static Pressure-Volume Curves

The *flexiVent system* can be used in studies that link tissue destruction with altered pulmonary function. Pressure-volume (PV) maneuvers can reliably measure the static compliance of the lung, which can increase significantly in models of emphysema and decrease after pneumonectomy and in models of acute lung injury or pulmonary fibrosis. PV loops capture the quasi-static mechanical properties of the respiratory system. The Salazar-Knowles equation can be fit to the expiratory branch of the PV loop, and quasi-static elastance and compliance values can be calculated. The commonly used outcomes in this analysis include: (1) A: this parameter represents the asymptote of the exponential function described by the Salazar-Knowles equation and estimates the subject's inspiratory capacity. (2) K: this parameter reflects the curvature of the upper portion of the deflation PV curve. (3) C_{st}: this parameter is the quasi-static compliance which reflects the static elastic recoil pressure of the lungs at a given lung volume. (4) Area: this parameter describes the area between the inflation and deflation limb of the PV curve. (5) PV curve: The comparative visual representation of PV curves can be very informative.

As with other perturbations, the animals need to be anesthetized, tracheotomized or orally intubated and then connected to the computer-controlled ventilator for mechanical ventilation. This analysis can often be performed in combination with other perturbations in an automated manner using a script. Shown in Fig. 5.3 is a PV curve acquired from a single control mouse in a stepwise manner. The outcomes derived from this analysis provide valuable information on the elastic properties of lung at baseline or in disease studies. Voltz et al. [37] reported that male mice had significantly higher basal quasi-static lung compliance than female mice and a more pronounced decline in static compliance after bleomycin administration. Since the data suggest that male C57BL/6 mice are more susceptible than female mice to bleomycin-induced lung function decline, a special attention to animals' sex, and genetic background would be advisable when designing experiments.

For the investigators who are interested in evaluating the inspiratory capacity while using the pneumonectomy model of lung regeneration, the deep lung inflation maneuver should be used instead of parameter A from the Salazar-Knowles equation to evaluate changes related to that specific lung volume. The reported values will more reliably reflect the corresponding pathologic changes because, at the difference of parameter A which offers an estimate of the inspiratory capacity from the Salazar-Knowles model, the deep lung inflation maneuver provides a direct and reliable measurement of that specific lung capacity.

Fig. 5.3 Example of a pressure-volume curve acquired in a mouse using a pressure-driven, stepwise approach. Starting from the end of an expiration, the lungs are gradually inflated to a pressure of 30 cmH2O in steps and then deflated in a similar manner

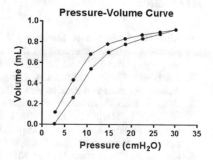

Application of in Vivo Invasive Analyses in Acute Lung Injury Studies

While the in vivo invasive analyses described above have been most widely applied in models of allergic airway disease [14, 20], they are also very useful in studies of models of COPD [25], pulmonary fibrosis [5, 33] and acute lung injury [1, 15]. The analyses mentioned above have been applied to studies of acute lung injury, where the pulmonary edema associated with that condition causes alveolar filling and dramatically affects the mechanical properties of the respiratory system. This is reflected by significant changes in C_{st}, R_{rs}, C_{rs}, or H. In mice challenged with LPS, Håkansson et al. [15] reported a 70 % decrease in C_{rs} and a 45 % increase in H at 48 h post-challenge relative to saline controls. By 96 h, all respiratory mechanics parameters had returned to baseline levels, with no significant difference compared with the time-matched saline controls.

Conclusion

Measuring lung function in mice is important to quantify functional abnormalities in models of common lung diseases and to evaluate the relevance of murine models to functional abnormalities that characterize human lung diseases such as asthma, COPD, acute lung injury, and pulmonary fibrosis. In this report, we shared our experience in performing such measurements in studies of lung disease models and provided practical details related to the use of the *flexiVent* in vivo invasive system in mice. Numerous studies [1, 4, 11, 21, 22, 25] have used this invasive approach to identify potentially useful therapeutic targets.

Acknowledgments The authors thank Dr. Xin Ren for assistance in lung function measurements, Dr. Dean Sheppard for helpful comments during the preparation of this chapter.

References

1. Allen GB, Cloutier ME, Larrabee YC, Tetenev K, Smiley ST, Bates JH. Neither fibrin nor plasminogen activator inhibitor-1 deficiency protects lung function in a mouse model of acute lung injury. Am J Physiol Lung Cell Mol Physiol. 2009;296(3):L277–85.
2. Baron RM, Choi AJ, Owen CA, Choi AM. Genetically manipulated mouse models of lung disease: potential and pitfalls. Am J Physiol Lung Cell Mol Physiol. 2012;302(6):L485–97.
3. Bates J, Irvin C, Brusasco V, Drazen J, Fredberg J, Loring S, Eidelman D, Ludwig M, Macklem P, Martin J, Milic-Emili J, Hantos Z, Hyatt R, Lai-Fook S, Leff A, Solway J, Lutchen K, Suki B, Mitzner W, Paré P, Pride N, Sly P. The use and misuse of Penh in animal models of lung disease. Am J Respir Cell Mol Biol. 2004;31(3):373–4.
4. Caceres AI, Brackmann M, Elia MD, Bessac BF, del Camino D, D'Amours M, Witek JS, Fanger CM, Chong JA, Hayward NJ, Homer RJ, Cohn L, Huang X, Moran MM, Jordt SE.

A sensory neuronal ion channel essential for airway inflammation and hyperreactivity in asthma. Proc Natl Acad Sci U.S.A. 2009;106(22):9099–104.

5. Card JW, Voltz JW, Carey MA, Bradbury JA, Degraff LM, Lih FB, Bonner JC, Morgan DL, Flake GP, Zeldin DC. Cyclooxygenase-2 deficiency exacerbates bleomycin-induced lung dysfunction but not fibrosis. Am J Respir Cell Mol Biol. 2007;37(3):300–8.

6. Cojocaru A, Irvin CG, Haverkamp HC, Bates JH. Computational assessment of airway wall stiffness in vivo in allergically inflamed mouse models of asthma. J Appl Physiol. (1985). 2008;104(6):1601–1610.

7. Cozzi E, Ackerman KG, Lundequist A, Drazen JM, Boyce JA, Beier DR. The naive airway hyperresponsiveness of the A/J mouse is Kit-mediated. Proc Natl Acad Sci USA. 2011;108 (31):12787–92.

8. De Sanctis GT, Merchant M, Beier DR, Dredge RD, Grobholz JK, Martin TR, Lander ES, Drazen JM. Quantitative locus analysis of airway hyperresponsiveness in A/J and C57BL/6 J mice. Nat Genet. 1995;11(2):150–4.

9. Drazen JM, Finn PW, De Sanctis GT. Mouse models of airway responsiveness: physiological basis of observed outcomes and analysis of selected examples using these outcome indicators. Annu Rev Physiol. 1999;61:593–625. Review.

10. Duguet A, Biyah K, Minshall E, Gomes R, Wang C-G, Taoudi-Benchekroun M, Bates JHT, Eidelman DH. Bronchial Responsiveness among Inbred Mouse Strains. Role of Airway Smooth-Muscle Shortening Velocity. Am J Respir Crit Care Med. 2000;161(3):839–48.

11. Egger C, Gérard C, Vidotto N, Accart N, Cannet C, Dunbar A, Tigani B, Piaia A, Jarai G, Jarman E, Schmid HA, Beckmann N. Lung volume quantified by MRI reflects extracellular-matrix deposition and altered pulmonary function in bleomycin models of fibrosis: effects of SOM230. Am J Physiol Lung Cell Mol Physiol. 2014;306(12):L1064–77.

12. Ferreira TP, de Arantes AC, do Nascimento CV, Olsen PC, Trentin PG, Rocco PR, Hogaboam CM, Puri RK, Martins MA, Silva PM. IL-13 immunotoxin accelerates resolution of lung pathological changes triggered by silica particles in mice. J Immunol. 2013;191 (10):5220–5229.

13. Glaab T, Taube C, Braun A, Mitzner W. Invasive and noninvasive methods for studying pulmonary function in mice. Respir Res. 2007;8:63. Review.

14. Grünig G, Warnock M, Wakil AE, Venkayya R, Brombacher F, Rennick DM, Sheppard D, Mohrs M, Donaldson DD, Locksley RM, Corry DB. Requirement for IL-13 independently of IL-4 in experimental asthma. Science. 1998;282(5397):2261–3.

15. Håkansson HF, Smailagic A, Brunmark C, Miller-Larsson A, Lal H. Altered lung function relates to inflammation in an acute LPS mouse model. Pulm Pharmacol Ther. 2012;25 (5):399–406.

16. Hamelmann E, Schwarze J, Takeda K, Oshiba A, Larsen GL, Irvin CG, Gelfand EW. Noninvasive measurement of airway responsiveness in allergic mice using barometric plethysmography. Am J Respir Crit Care Med. 1997;156(3 Pt 1):766–75.

17. Hantos Z, Daroczy B, Suki B, Nagy S, Fredberg JJ. Input impedance and peripheral inhomogeneity in dog lungs. J Appl Physiol. 1992;72(1):168–78.

18. Jucker M. The benefits and limitations of animal models for translational research in neurodegenerative diseases. Nat Med. 2010;16(11):1210–4.

19. Kearley J, Erjefalt JS, Andersson C, Benjamin E, Jones CP, Robichaud A, Pegorier S, Brewah Y, Burwell TJ, Bjermer L, Kiener PA, Kolbeck R, Lloyd CM, Coyle AJ, Humbles AA. IL-9 governs allergen-induced mast cell numbers in the lung and chronic remodeling of the airways. Am J Respir Crit Care Med. 2011;183(7):865–75.

20. Köhl J, Baelder R, Lewkowich IP, Pandey MK, Hawlisch H, Wang L, Best J, Herman NS, Sproles AA, Zwirner J, Whitsett JA, Gerard C, Sfyroera G, Lambris JD, Wills-Karp M. A regulatory role for the C5a anaphylatoxin in type 2 immunity in asthma. J Clin Invest. 2006;116(3):783–96.

21. Kudo M, Melton AC, Chen C, Engler MB, Huang KE, Ren X, Wang Y, Bernstein X, Li JT, Atabai K, Huang X*, Sheppard D. IL-17A produced by αβ T cells drives airway

hyper-responsiveness in mice and enhances mouse and human airway smooth muscle contraction. Nat Med. 2012;18(4):547–54.

22. Kuperman DA, Huang XZ, Koth LL, Chang GH, Dolganov GM, Zhu Z, Elias JA, Sheppard D, Erle DJ. Direct effects of interleukin-13 on epithelial cells cause airway hyperreactivity and mucus overproduction in asthma. Nat Med. 2002;8:885–9.

23. Lovgren AK, Jania LA, Hartney JM, Parsons KK, Audoly LP, Fitzgerald GA, Tilley SL, Koller BH. COX-2-derived prostacyclin protects against bleomycin-induced pulmonary fibrosis. Am J Physiol Lung Cell Mol Physiol. 2006;291(2):L144–56.

24. McGovern TK, Robichaud A, Fereydoonzad L, Schuessler TF, Martin JG. Evaluation of respiratory system mechanics in mice using the forced oscillation technique. J Vis Exp. 2013;75:e50172. doi:10.3791/50172.

25. Mouded M, Egea EE, Brown MJ, Hanlon SM, Houghton AM, Tsai LW, Ingenito EP, Shapiro SD. Epithelial cell apoptosis causes acute lung injury masquerading as emphysema. Am J Respir Cell Mol Biol. 2009;41(4):407–14.

26. North ML, Amatullah H, Khanna N, Urch B, Grasemann H, Silverman F, Scott JA. Augmentation of arginase 1 expression by exposure to air pollution exacerbates the airways hyperresponsiveness in murine models of asthma. Respir Res. 2011;12(1):19.

27. Orme J Jr, Romney JS, Hopkins RO, Pope D, Chan KJ, Thomsen G, Crapo RO, Weaver LK, Pulmonary function and health-related quality of life in survivors of acute respiratory distress syndrome. Am J Respir Crit Care Med. 2003;167(5):690–694.

28. Peták F, Habre W, Donati YR, Hantos Z, Barazzone-Argiroffo C, Hyperoxia-induced changes in mouse lung mechanics: forced oscillations vs. barometric plethysmography. J Appl Physiol. (1985). 2001;90(6):2221–2230.

29. Rao S, Verkman AS. Analysis of organ physiology in transgenic mice. Am J Physiol Cell Physiol. 2000;279(1):C1–18.

30. Robichaud A, Fereydoonzad L, Urovitch IB, Brunet JD. Comparative study of three *flexiVent* system configurations using mechanical test loads. Exp Lung Res. 2014. doi:10.3109/01902148.2014.971921 (Epub ahead of print).

31. Shalaby KH, Gold LG, Schuessler TF, Martin JG, Robichaud A. Combined forced oscillation and forced expiration measurements in mice for the assessment of airway hyperresponsiveness. Respir Res. 2010;11:82.

32. Suzukawa M, Morita H, Nambu A, Arae K, Shimura E, Shibui A, Yamaguchi S, Suzukawa K, Nakanishi W, Oboki K, Kajiwara N, Ohno T, Ishii A, Körner H, Cua DJ, Suto H, Yoshimoto T, Iwakura Y, Yamasoba T, Ohta K, Sudo K, Saito H, Okumura K, Broide DH, Matsumoto K, Nakae S. Epithelial cell-derived IL-25, but not Th17 cell-derived IL-17 or IL-17F, is crucial for murine asthma. J Immunol. 2012;189(7):3641–52 Epub 2012 Aug 31.

33. Tanaka K-I, Azuma A, Sato K, Mizushima T. Effects of lecithinized superoxide dismutase and/or pirfenidone against bleomycin-induced pulmonary fibrosis. Chest. 2012;142(4):1011–9.

34. Tomioka S, Bates JH, Irvin CG. Airway and tissue mechanics in a murine model of asthma: alveolar capsule vs. forced oscillations. J Appl Physiol. (1985). 2002;93(1):263–70.

35. Wong PC, Cai H, Borchelt DR, Price DL. Genetically engineered mouse models of neurodegenerative diseases. Nat Neurosci. 2002;5(7):633–9.

36. Vanoirbeek JA, Rinaldi M, De Vooght V, Haenen S, Bobic S, Gayan-Ramirez G, Hoet PH, Verbeken E, Decramer M, Nemery B, Janssens W. Noninvasive and invasive pulmonary function in mouse models of obstructive and restrictive respiratory diseases. Am J Respir Cell Mol Biol. 2010;42(1):96–104.

37. Voltz JW, Card JW, Carey MA, DeGraff LM, Ferguson CD, Flake GP, Bonner JC, Korach KS, Zeldin DC. Male sex hormones exacerbate lung function impairment after bleomycin-induced pulmonary fibrosis. Am J Respir Cell Mol Biol. 2008;39(1):45–52.

38. Zheng T, Zhu Z, Wang Z, Homer RJ, Ma B, Riese RJ Jr, Chapman HA Jr, Shapiro SD, Elias JA. Inducible targeting of IL-13 to the adult lung causes matrix metalloproteinase- and cathepsin-dependent emphysema. J Clin Invest. 2000;106(9):1081–93.

Chapter 6
Analysis of Epithelial Injury and Repair

Kathrin Mutze and Melanie Königshoff

Abbreviations

α-SMA	Alpha smooth muscle actin
ALI	Acute lung injury
ABCA3	ATP-binding cassette sub-family A member 3
AQP5	Aquaporin 5
ATI	Alveolar epithelial type I cell
ATII	Alveolar epithelial type II cell
BMP	Bone morphogenetic protein
BrdU	Bromodeoxyuridine
COPD	Chronic obstructive pulmonary disease
ECAD	E-cadherin, epithelial cadherin
ECM	Extracellular matrix
EGFP	Enhanced green fluorescent protein
EMT	Epithelial-to-mesenchymal transition
EpCAM	Epithelial cell adhesion molecule
GFP	Green fluorescent protein
FACS	Fluorescence Activated Cell Sorting
IPF	Idiopathic pulmonary fibrosis
KGF	Keratinocyte growth factor
LAMP3	Lysosome-associated membrane glycoprotein 3
PARP	Poly (ADP-ribose) polymerase
RAGE	Receptor for advanced glycosylation end products
SPA	Surfactant protein A
SPB	Surfactant protein B
SPC	Surfactant protein C
SPD	Surfactant protein D
TGF-β	Transforming growth factor beta

K. Mutze · M. Königshoff (✉)
Comprehensive Pneumology Center (CPC), Helmholtz Zentrum Munich and
Ludwig-Maximilians-University Munich, Max-Lebsche-Platz 31, 81377 Munich, Germany
e-mail: melanie.koenigshoff@helmholtz-muenchen.de

© Springer International Publishing AG 2017
L.M. Schnapp and C. Feghali-Bostwick (eds.), *Acute Lung Injury and Repair*,
Respiratory Medicine, DOI 10.1007/978-3-319-46527-2_6

69

T1α   Podoplanin
TJ   Tight junctions
TJP1   Tight junction protein 1
TUNEL   TdT-mediated dUTP-biotin nick end labeling
WNT   Wingless-type MMTV integration site family member

Introduction

Acute and chronic lung diseases constitute a significant health burden worldwide and a better and deeper understanding of the mechanisms that initiate and drive disease progression [1–3]. Alveolar epithelial injury represents a hallmark of acute lung injury (ALI) as well as chronic lung diseases such as idiopathic pulmonary fibrosis (IPF) and chronic obstructive pulmonary disease (COPD) [1, 4, 5]. In the healthy adult lung, alveolar epithelial type I (ATI) and alveolar epithelial type II (ATII) cells are the main cell types that form the alveolar epithelium and establish the alveolar epithelial barrier [6]. ATI cells represent large, thin squamous epithelial cells that cover an enormous surface area (95 % of the alveolus) and are in close vicinity to the underlying capillary endothelium to facilitate gas exchange [7–9]. ATII cells, however, display a cuboidal shape and one of their main functions is the production, storage and release of surfactant. Surfactant consists of an intricate combination of proteins and lipids which lines the alveolar epithelium, lowers the surface tension in the lung and plays an important role in host defense mechanisms [10, 11]. Both ATI and ATII cells participate in ion transport in the lung and contribute to the fluid balance within the alveolus [7, 12, 13]. In ALI, the alveolar epithelial barrier, formed by ATI and ATII cells as well as endothelial cells of the alveolar capillary, represents the first point of injury. Disruption of the barrier structure with subsequent accumulation of protein-rich edema fluid in the alveolar air spaces is a main feature of ALI [14–16]. Tight junctions (TJ) localizing to the cell–cell junctions connecting alveolar epithelial cells are essential for normal epithelial barrier function [17]. ATII cells are a critical cell population driving repair in the alveolar epithelium [18]. ATII cells are able to proliferate, self-renew and serve as a progenitor cell population for ATI cells in injury and repair processes induced by a variety of different triggers. Thus, ATII cells are considered one of the important epithelial stem cell populations in the adult distal lung [19–22]. Restoration of the normal epithelial barrier requires the spreading and migration of cells in close proximity to the injury to cover the denuded basement membrane. This is followed by migration and proliferation of progenitor cells to compensate for the cellular loss. Finally differentiation processes have to be initiated to restore a functional epithelium [14, 23, 24]. However, the loss of reparative function of ATII cells and a shift towards pro-fibrotic functions has been described for ALI as well as for IPF [25–29]. The elucidation of mechanisms driving alveolar epithelial cell responses in a beneficial versus a potentially detrimental direction during lung injury and repair is therefore of prime interest and the development of novel models and methods to study those mechanisms is of utmost importance.

Methods of Alveolar Epithelial Type II Cell Isolation

A prerequisite for analyzing alveolar epithelial type II cell characteristics and functional properties in vitro is the isolation of a pure population of the respective primary cell type. This requires the identification of specific ATII cell markers within the tissue together with morphology and localization. Several markers expressed in adult ATII cells have been described over the past decades. These include the surfactant proteins A, B, C, and D (SPA, SPB, SPC, and SPD), of which SPC has been reported to be specific for ATII cells [30]. ATII specific expression of ATP-binding cassette sub-family A member 3 (ABCA3), a membrane component of lamellar bodies [31], in which surfactant proteins are stored [32], has been reported. In addition, lysosome-associated membrane glycoprotein 3 (LAMP3) [33] and pepsinogen C [34] have been proposed as ATII markers. Immunization strategies by Boylan [35] and Gonzalez [36] used ATII cells as immunogens to generate monoclonal antibodies for ATII cell surface proteins for rat and human. The monoclonal antibody MMC4 recognized a novel antigen on the apical surface of rat ATII cells, but also bound to rat club cells [35]. An antibody generated against human ATII cells recognized a protein of 280- to 300-kDa on the apical plasma membrane, which was termed HTII-280 and, by analysis of its biochemical characteristics, represents an integral membrane protein [36].

Two main isolation strategies have been widely used to isolate ATII cells from rodent and human tissue. Both strategies share a common procedure of enzymatic dissociation of lung tissue to obtain a single cell suspension of the lung. Enzymes most frequently used include porcine elastase, dispase, or collagenase as well as different combinations thereof [37–40]. In case of the murine lung, enzymes are directly instilled into the parenchyma via the cannulated trachea [38]. In case of human tissue, direct instillation into the alveolar region via a bronchus can only be applied for closed lung segments [28, 39]. Alternatively, minced human distal lung tissue can be subjected to enzymatic digestion [40]. Following digestion, alveolar tissue is dissected from the lager airways and minced mechanically. After sequential filtration of cells through nylon meshes of different pore sizes ranging from 100 to 10 μm to obtain a single cell suspension [38, 39], ATII cells can be isolated via positive or negative selection or a combinatorial approach making use of positive as well as negative selection markers.

Several different separation methods can be applied subsequently using different marker combinations. The most commonly used methods for depletion of specific subset of cells include the use of antibody coated cell culture plates, where cells expressing the respective markers adhere to the plate and non-adherent cells are collected [41–43], or using antibodies coupled to magnetic beads [38, 44, 45], and similarly the non-bound cells are collected.

Antibodies directed against CD45, CD14, and CD16/32 for hematopoietic lineages such macrophages, neutrophils and lymphocytes are commonly used [21, 27, 38, 43, 45–47] for negative selection. Species-specific IgG antibodies binding with their Fc domain to the Fcγ-receptors on the cell surface of phagocytes, B-lymphocytes, natural killer cells and dendritic cells are also widely used to eliminate these cell populations from the preparation [41–43, 45, 48–50]. Depletion of CD31 positive endothelial cells is often included in different protocols [44]. Furthermore, a fluorescence activated cell sorting (FACS) based approach can be utilized by using fluorescently labeled antibodies and subsequent sorting of cells, displaying no positive signal for any of the utilized markers [51]. Isolation protocols applied for human ATII cells frequently contain previous enrichment of ATII cells for the downstream depletion strategy by subjecting the crude singe cell suspension after enzymatic digestion to a discontinuous Percoll density gradient (1.04–1.09 g/ml). After centrifugation ATII cells and macrophages will be found in the same layer of the Percoll gradient. The cells in this layer can be isolated and subsequently a depletion of alveolar macrophages can be performed [41, 42, 45].

Positive selection strategies are mainly applied for the isolation of lineage labeled ATII cells in murine mouse models by FACS. For this strategy SPC-driver lines are used, which express GFP or EGFP under the control of the SPC promoter [7, 52–54]. In this context, it has been shown that transgenic mice exhibiting GFP expression under the control of the human SPC promoter in the murine system display GFP expression in only a subset of ATII cells or additionally in bronchiolar epithelial cells [55, 56]. However, the use of murine SPC promoters was reported to generate a higher specificity of labeling ATII cells [52, 53] although the efficiency of labeling was also described to be dependent on the age of mice [52] and isolated ATII cell displayed some heterogeneity as cells with bronchiolar and alveolar epithelial gene signatures were detected under three-dimensional culture conditions [52]. The positive selection of human ATII cells by FACS using an antibody against the previously described HTII-280 membrane protein has been initially described by Gonzalez and colleagues [36].

Combined negative and positive selection strategies are applied using different combinations of negative depletion for of a variety of cell types, and are listed in Table 6.1. These markers include markers for cells from hematopoietic lineages [22, 28, 40, 57–60], and ATI cells (T1α positive cells) [40] and a positive selection for general epithelial markers such as EpCAM [22, 40, 57, 59–61] and E-cadherin [28, 58] or a lysosomal marker such as the fluorescent dye LysoTracker [59], labeling acidic organelles within live cells.

Overall, the different ATII cell isolation strategies result in some variability of cell purity (between 80 and 99 %). The choice of the appropriate isolation method is widely discussed in particular with respect to the utilization for the isolation of ATII cells from different models of lung disease or the subsequent usage of cells for different downstream applications (direct analysis versus culture for functional assays). When choosing which methods to apply, several points need to be taken under consideration. In general, the use of positive selection markers might result in higher cell purity—and better characterized cell (sub)populations, however, changes

Table 6.1 Markers for the depletion or enrichment of specific cell populations

	Marker	Targeted cell population	Reference
Negative selection *Depletion of unwanted cell populations*	CD45	Differentiated hematopoietic cells, except erythrocytes and platelets	[22, 27, 28, 38]
	CD16/32	Macrophages, monocytes, B-cells, NK cells, neutrophils, mast cells, dendritic cells	[38, 44, 46]
	CD11c	Macrophages, monocytes, NK cells, dendritic cells, granulocytes, subsets of B- and T-cells	[51]
	CD11b	Macrophages, monocytes, NK cells, dendritic cells, granulocytes, subsets of B- and T-cell	[51]
	F4/80	Macrophages	[51]
	CD14	Macrophages, monocytes, dendritic cells, granulocytes	[45, 60]
	CD19	B-cells, follicular dendritic cells	[51]
	CD31	Endothelial cells	[44]
	T1α	Alveolar epithelial type I cells	[40]
Positive selection *Enrichment for wanted cell population*	HTII-280	Alveolar epithelial type II cells	[22, 36]
	EpCAM	Epithelial cells	[22, 40, 59–61]
	ECAD	Epithelial cells	[28]
	SPC-GFP	SPC expressing alveolar epithelial type II cells and bronchiolar epithelial cells (lineage–labeled)	[28, 52, 53, 56]
	LysoTracker	Lysosomal rich cells	[59]

in the expression pattern of single specific markers used for selection might be altered in different disease models, which in turn changes the population analyzed.

Alveolar Epithelial Type II Cell Analysis

Obtaining insight into molecular mechanisms of alveolar epithelial injury and repair is of prime interest to identified potential targets for therapeutic intervention needed for the treatment of various lung diseases, including ARDS.

Alveolar Epithelial Type II Cell Culture

Analyzing freshly isolated ATII cells from rodent injury models or human diseased tissue using microarray technology is a powerful tool to determine disease related altered phenotypes in lung injury and repair [27, 40]. However, for functional analysis, the culture of primary ATII cells is of utmost importance. Challenged by the fact that ATII cells possess the intrinsic properties to differentiate into ATI cells when placed into normal cell culture, a wide range of culture conditions and media compositions for ATII cells are described. A careful selection of culture conditions is crucial to obtain meaningful results. Depending on the applied assay, culture vessels as well as the presence of specific media supplements might influence experimental outcomes. Plating fresh ATII cells on plastic dishes induces the gradual loss of ATII cell characteristic [62, 63]. Coating cell culture dishes with extracellular matrix (ECM) components such as fibronectin, collagen or laminin or a combination thereof, will lead to differences in the dynamics of trans-differentiation processes. Additionally, culturing of ATII cells on trans-well filter inserts has been described to result in stabilized monolayers of ATII cells and allow cultures at the air liquid interphase [61]. Furthermore, the supplementation of commonly used cell culture media (e.g., DMEM or DMEM/F12) with KGF [64–67] and glucocorticoids in the combination with cAMP [68, 69] has been described to promote ATII cell phenotype in culture.

Alveolar Epithelial Type II Cell Proliferation

Due to their role as progenitor cells, the proliferative capacity of ATII cells is a critical feature in lung injury and repair processes within the lung. Thus, the assessment of proliferative behavior of this cell population is one of the most assessed cell characteristics. For the determination of in vitro proliferation capacity several different methods can be applied. Determination of gene and protein expression of genes related to cell cycle progression such as Ki67, Ccng1, and Ccng2 [27], are widely used to compare proliferative capacities of injured versus non-injured ATII cells and furthermore their response to different stimuli. The analysis of protein expression of proliferation markers Ki67 [27, 70], PCNA [71, 72] and phosphorylated histone H3 [27, 73] in cells in vitro as well as in in vivo models by immunofluorescence/immunohistochemistry represents a complementary approach. Direct functional assays for the detection of proliferating cells include the use of metabolic activity assays such as the WST-1 assay [74, 75] where a tetrazolium salt is converted in a colored formazan by endogenous dehydrogenates displaying a proportional relationship to cell number. Furthermore, the incorporation of bromodeoxyuridine (BrdU) [21] or [3H]thymidine [27] into the DNA of proliferating cells represents the gold standard for determining proliferation. Usage of several of these techniques provided insight in the reprogrammed phenotype and aberrant proliferative capacity of fibrotic ATII cells and the observation that targeting this phenotype attenuates pulmonary fibrosis in different models [27, 70].

Alveolar Epithelial Type II Cell Apoptosis

Besides changes in the proliferative behavior of injured ATII cells, the presence of apoptosis is another important parameter when analyzing injury and repair processes in the lung epithelium. The most commonly applied strategies are the analysis of caspase activity [76, 77] and the caspase mediated cleavage of endogenous substrates such as PARP [77], a crucial step in the apoptotic process. Furthermore, early apoptotic changes such as the flip of phosphatidylserine from the inside to the outside of the cell plasma membrane is used as a surrogate marker for apoptosis and detected by Annexin V binding and further analysis by flow cytometry [77]. TdT-mediated dUTP-biotin nick end labeling (TUNEL), a method to detect DNA fragmentation occurring in apoptotic cells, can be used for in vitro studies as well as for the detection of apoptotic cells in tissues of in vivo models of lung injury [70, 78]. The use of TUNEL staining provided data on the presence of increased numbers of apoptotic alveolar epithelial cells in fibrotic mouse models, as well as IPF tissue [70, 78, 79].

Epithelial to Mesenchymal Transition (EMT) of ATII Cells

Besides the described imbalance of proliferation and apoptosis in models of epithelial injury, the occurrence of EMT is widely discussed in the context of attempted alveolar repair processes. In vitro studies of EMT of cultured epithelial cells regularly use the cytokine TGF-β1 for EMT induction, which has been demonstrated in several organs including the lung [80–82]. Monitoring of decreased expression of epithelial marker genes such as E-Cadherin, cytokeratin and TJ-proteins is performed for the characterization of epithelial integrity on gene expression level as well as on protein level. Moreover, analysis should include the expression of EMT transcription factors, such as Snail, Slug, Zeb, or Twist as well as mesenchymal markers. Several mesenchymal markers, including αSMA, Calponin, and ECM related proteins such as collagen1, fibronectin and vimentin are used to describe the gain of mesenchymal cell characteristics [27, 80, 83, 84]. Importantly, co-expression of epithelial and mesenchymal markers by immunofluorescence/immunohistochemistry staining should be analyzed and has been demonstrated in human tissue of different lung diseases [28, 85, 86]. These descriptive investigations should be further complemented with functional cell assays, such as cell migration, which is a prominent feature of EMT.

For studying the in vivo relevance of findings generated by in vitro cultures, lineage tracing animals can be used to determine the cell fate in the context of lung injury. These studies utilize different transgene mouse strains, which express traceable markers under the control of the surfactant protein C promotor [19, 86, 87].

Alveolar Epithelial Trans-Differentiation

ATII cells expressing surfactant proteins are able to self-renew and trans-differentiate into ATI cells [20, 22, 88–90]. Depending on the type of injury applied, other epithelial cell populations, negative for SPC, can contribute to the attenuation of lung injury [58, 91]. Therefore, understanding how ATII cells differentiate into an ATI cell phenotype is under intense investigation including respective gene expression signatures as well as the morphological conversion from a cuboidal to a squamous cell shape. Early studies described the trans-differentiation of ATII cells into ATI-like cells in primary culture. These observations were based on the gradual loss of gene and protein expression of surfactant proteins as well as the loss of lamellar bodies, investigated by the use of electron microscopy [92]. Furthermore, the gain of features of ATI cells such as a flattened cell morphology and the expression of ATI cell-associated markers T1α (podoplanin) [93–96], aquaporin 5 (AQP5) [64, 97], receptor for advanced glycosylation end products (RAGE), and caveolin [98–100] were described. An overview of ATII and ATI cell specific markers is displayed in Table 6.2. Applying freshly isolated ATII cells to standard cell culture conditions is now widely used to mimic differentiation and repair mechanisms to investigate molecular cues in response to lung injury. The model has been utilized to study ATII cell trans-differentiation potential in various species including rat, mouse and human. Monitoring of epithelial cell identity and trans-differentiation is mainly achieved by gene and protein expression analysis of the respective markers in combination with microscopic evaluation of cell morphology.

Utilizing the spontaneous trans-differentiation of primary ATII cells in culture shed light into molecular programs that regulate this process and identified essential developmental pathways, such as the Wnt/β-catenin pathway [47, 60, 96, 103, 104] as well as TGF-β and BMP signaling [46, 105] to be involved.

However, it has to be taken into account that the model of ATII to ATI cell trans-differentiation in vitro does not fully resemble the processes occurring in vivo, as the specific trigger of injury has been shown to modulate a differential response of ATII and other progenitor cell populations. Furthermore, data indicate that the expression profile of freshly isolated ATI cells does not completely concur with the profile of ATI-like cells derived from trans-differentiation models in vitro [106].

Table 6.2 ATII versus ATI cell markers/characteristics for the determination of trans-differentiation

	Marker/characteristics	Reference
ATII cells	SPC	[30, 96]
	ABCA3	[31]
	LAMP3	[33]
ATI/AT1-like cells	T1α	[93–95]
	AQP5	[64, 97]
	HOPX	[22, 101]
	RAGE	[96, 102]
	Caveolin-1	[98–100]

To overcome the limitations of 2D cell culture models for studying ATII to ATI trans-differentiation and the regenerative potential of the ATII cell progenitor pool, the establishment of new 3D culture methods has been expedited extensively [22, 107], comparably to strategies for the generation of 3D organoids from colon, small intestine, and stomach [108]. For the purpose of mimicking the 3D microenvironment of the lung alveolus, primary ATII cells are seeded as a single cell suspension in an ECM mixture which is secreted by Engelbreth-Holm-Swarm (EHS) mouse sarcoma cells (Matrigel), [22, 109]. Studies utilizing the co-culture of ATII cells with other cell populations such as fibroblasts or endothelial cells in matrigel describe the formation of lung organoids which display cuboidal ATII cells expressing SPC on the outer layer of the organoid. The organoid lumen, however, is lined by thin, squamous epithelial cells expressing markers of differentiated ATI cells such as AQP5 and T1α, indicating a self-renewal as well as a trans-differentiation capacity of ATII cells in this setting, and therefore representing an advanced model for studying mechanisms involved in this process in a more in vivo-related fashion [22, 101].

Short Summary

Alveolar epithelial cells play a crucial role in lung injury and repair processes in response to different stimuli and in the context of various lung diseases. A careful characterization of specific disease related alveolar epithelial phenotypes using comprehensive approaches and improved culturing methodologies will lead to important insights into novel therapeutic strategies targeting lung injury and repair.

References

1. Bhattacharya J, Matthay MA. Regulation and repair of the alveolar-capillary barrier in acute lung injury. Annu Rev Physiol. 2013;75:593–615 (Epub 2013/02/13).
2. Fernandez IE, Eickelberg O. New cellular and molecular mechanisms of lung injury and fibrosis in idiopathic pulmonary fibrosis. Lancet. 2012;380(9842):680–8 (Epub 2012/08/21).
3. Barnes PJ. Cellular and molecular mechanisms of chronic obstructive pulmonary disease. Clin Chest Med. 2014;35(1):71–86 (Epub 2014/02/11).
4. Thorley AJ, Tetley TD. Pulmonary epithelium, cigarette smoke, and chronic obstructive pulmonary disease. Int J Chronic Obstr Pulm Dis. 2007;2(4):409–28 (Epub 2008/02/14).
5. Selman M, Pardo A. Role of epithelial cells in idiopathic pulmonary fibrosis: from innocent targets to serial killers. Proc Am Thorac Soc. 2006;3(4):364–72 (Epub 2006/06/02).
6. Dobbs LG, Johnson MD. Alveolar epithelial transport in the adult lung. Respir Physiol Neurobiol. 2007;159(3):283–300 (Epub 2007/08/11).
7. Dobbs LG, Johnson MD, Vanderbilt J, Allen L, Gonzalez R. The great big alveolar TI cell: evolving concepts and paradigms. Cellular Physiol Biochem Int J Exp Cell Physiol Biochem Pharmacol. 2010;25(1):55–62 (Epub 2010/01/08).

8. Crapo JD, Barry BE, Gehr P, Bachofen M, Weibel ER. Cell number and cell characteristics of the normal human lung. Am Rev Respir Dis. 1982;126(2):332–7 (Epub 1982/08/01).
9. Weibel ER. On the tricks alveolar epithelial cells play to make a good lung. Am J Respir Crit Care Med. 2015;191(5):504–13 (Epub 2015/02/28).
10. Fehrenbach H. Alveolar epithelial type II cell: defender of the alveolus revisited. Respir Res. 2001;2(1):33–46 (Epub 2001/11/01).
11. Mulugeta S, Beers MF. Surfactant protein C: its unique properties and emerging immunomodulatory role in the lung. Microbes and infection/Institut Pasteur. 2006;8 (8):2317–23 (Epub 2006/06/20).
12. Eaton DC, Helms MN, Koval M, Bao HF, Jain L. The contribution of epithelial sodium channels to alveolar function in health and disease. Annu Rev Physiol. 2009;71:403–23 (Epub 2008/10/04).
13. Kim KJ, Malik AB. Protein transport across the lung epithelial barrier. Am J Physiol Lung Cell Mol Physiol. 2003;284(2):L247–59 (Epub 2003/01/21).
14. Ware LB, Matthay MA. The acute respiratory distress syndrome. N Eng J Med. 2000;342 (18):1334–49 (Epub 2000/05/04).
15. Pugin J, Verghese G, Widmer MC, Matthay MA. The alveolar space is the site of intense inflammatory and profibrotic reactions in the early phase of acute respiratory distress syndrome. Crit Care Med. 1999;27(2):304–12 (Epub 1999/03/13).
16. Johnson ER, Matthay MA. Acute lung injury: epidemiology, pathogenesis, and treatment. J Aerosol Med Pulm Drug Deliv. 2010;23(4):243–52 (Epub 2010/01/16).
17. Koval M. Tight junctions, but not too tight: fine control of lung permeability by claudins. Am J Physiol Lung Cell Mol Physiol. 2009;297(2):L217–8 (Epub 2009/06/16).
18. Hogan BL, Barkauskas CE, Chapman HA, Epstein JA, Jain R, Hsia CC, et al. Repair and regeneration of the respiratory system: complexity, plasticity, and mechanisms of lung stem cell function. Cell Stem Cell. 2014;15(2):123–38 (Epub 2014/08/12).
19. Rock JR, Barkauskas CE, Cronce MJ, Xue Y, Harris JR, Liang J, et al. Multiple stromal populations contribute to pulmonary fibrosis without evidence for epithelial to mesenchymal transition. Proc Natl Acad Sci USA. 2011;108(52):E1475–83 (Epub 2011/11/30).
20. Desai TJ, Brownfield DG, Krasnow MA. Alveolar progenitor and stem cells in lung development, renewal and cancer. Nature. 2014;507(7491):190–4 (Epub 2014/02/07).
21. Liu Y, Sadikot RT, Adami GR, Kalinichenko VV, Pendyala S, Natarajan V, et al. FoxM1 mediates the progenitor function of type II epithelial cells in repairing alveolar injury induced by Pseudomonas aeruginosa. J Exp Med. 2011;208(7):1473–84 (Epub 2011/06/29).
22. Barkauskas CE, Cronce MJ, Rackley CR, Bowie EJ, Keene DR, Stripp BR, et al. Type 2 alveolar cells are stem cells in adult lung. J Clin Investig. 2013;123(7):3025–36 (Epub 2013/08/08).
23. Crosby LM, Waters CM. Epithelial repair mechanisms in the lung. Am J Physiol Lung Cell Mol Physiol. 2010;298(6):L715–31 (Epub 2010/04/07).
24. Zahm JM, Kaplan H, Herard AL, Doriot F, Pierrot D, Somelette P, et al. Cell migration and proliferation during the in vitro wound repair of the respiratory epithelium. Cell Motil Cytoskelet. 1997;37(1):33–43 (Epub 1997/01/01).
25. Bitterman PB. Pathogenesis of fibrosis in acute lung injury. Am J Med. 1992;92(6A):39S–43S (Epub 1992/06/22).
26. Sapru A, Flori H, Quasney MW, Dahmer MK. Pathobiology of acute respiratory distress syndrome. Pediatr Crit Care Med J Soc Crit Care Med World Fed Pediatr Intensive Crit Care Soc. 2015;16(5 Suppl 1):S6–22 (Epub 2015/06/03).
27. Königshoff M, Kramer M, Balsara N, Wilhelm J, Amarie OV, Jahn A, et al. WNT1-inducible signaling protein-1 mediates pulmonary fibrosis in mice and is upregulated in humans with idiopathic pulmonary fibrosis. J Clin Investig. 2009;119(4):772–87 (Epub 2009/03/17).
28. Marmai C, Sutherland RE, Kim KK, Dolganov GM, Fang X, Kim SS, et al. Alveolar epithelial cells express mesenchymal proteins in patients with idiopathic pulmonary fibrosis. Am J Physiol Lung Cell Mol Physiol. 2011;301(1):L71–8 (Epub 2011/04/19).

29. Aumiller V, Balsara N, Wilhelm J, Gunther A, Königshoff M. WNT/β-catenin signaling induces IL-1β expression by alveolar epithelial cells in pulmonary fibrosis. Am J Respir Cell Mol Biol. 2013;49(1):96–104 (Epub 2013/03/26).

30. Kuroki Y, Voelker DR. Pulmonary surfactant proteins. J Biol Chem. 1994;269(42):25943–6 (Epub 1994/10/21).

31. Yamano G, Funahashi H, Kawanami O, Zhao LX, Ban N, Uchida Y, et al. ABCA3 is a lamellar body membrane protein in human lung alveolar type II cells. FEBS Lett. 2001;508 (2):221–5 (Epub 2001/11/24).

32. Schmitz G, Muller G. Structure and function of lamellar bodies, lipid-protein complexes involved in storage and secretion of cellular lipids. J Lipid Res. 1991;32(10):1539–70 (Epub 1991/10/01).

33. Salaun B, de Saint-Vis B, Pacheco N, Pacheco Y, Riesler A, Isaac S, et al. CD208/dendritic cell-lysosomal associated membrane protein is a marker of normal and transformed type II pneumocytes. Am J Pathol. 2004;164(3):861–71 (Epub 2004/02/26).

34. Foster C, Aktar A, Kopf D, Zhang P, Guttentag S. Pepsinogen C: a type 2 cell-specific protease. Am J Physiol Lung Cell Mol Physiol. 2004;286(2):L382–7 (Epub 2003/10/28).

35. Boylan GM, Pryde JG, Dobbs LG, McElroy MC. Identification of a novel antigen on the apical surface of rat alveolar epithelial type II and Clara cells. Am J Physiol Lung Cell Mol Physiol. 2001;280(6):L1318–26 (Epub 2001/05/15).

36. Gonzalez RF, Allen L, Gonzales L, Ballard PL, Dobbs LG. HTII-280, a biomarker specific to the apical plasma membrane of human lung alveolar type II cells. J Histochem Cytochem Off J Histochem Soc. 2010;58(10):891–901 (Epub 2010/06/23).

37. Dobbs LG, Gonzalez R, Williams MC. An improved method for isolating type II cells in high yield and purity. Am Rev Respir Dis. 1986;134(1):141–5 (Epub 1986/07/01).

38. Corti M, Brody AR, Harrison JH. Isolation and primary culture of murine alveolar type II cells. Am J Respir Cell Mol Biol. 1996;14(4):309–15 (Epub 1996/04/01).

39. Frank J, Roux J, Kawakatsu H, Su G, Dagenais A, Berthiaume Y, et al. Transforming growth factor-β1 decreases expression of the epithelial sodium channel αENaC and alveolar epithelial vectorial sodium and fluid transport via an ERK1/2-dependent mechanism. J Biol Chem. 2003;278(45):43939–50 (Epub 2003/08/22).

40. Fujino N, Kubo H, Ota C, Suzuki T, Suzuki S, Yamada M, et al. A novel method for isolating individual cellular components from the adult human distal lung. Am J Respir Cell Mol Biol. 2012;46(4):422–30 (Epub 2011/10/29).

41. Ballard PL, Lee JW, Fang X, Chapin C, Allen L, Segal MR, et al. Regulated gene expression in cultured type II cells of adult human lung. Am J Physiol Lung Cell Mol Physiol. 2010;299 (1):L36–50 (Epub 2010/04/13).

42. Fang X, Song Y, Hirsch J, Galietta LJ, Pedemonte N, Zemans RL, et al. Contribution of CFTR to apical-basolateral fluid transport in cultured human alveolar epithelial type II cells. Am J Physiol Lung Cell Mol Physiol. 2006;290(2):L242–9 (Epub 2005/09/07).

43. Chen J, Chen Z, Narasaraju T, Jin N, Liu L. Isolation of highly pure alveolar epithelial type I and type II cells from rat lungs. Laboratory investigation; a journal of technical methods and pathology. 2004;84(6):727–35 (Epub 2004/04/13).

44. Unkel B, Hoegner K, Clausen BE, Lewe-Schlosser P, Bodner J, Gattenloehner S, et al. Alveolar epithelial cells orchestrate DC function in murine viral pneumonia. J Clin Investig. 2012;122(10):3652–64 (Epub 2012/09/22).

45. Mao P, Wu S, Li J, Fu W, He W, Liu X, et al. Human alveolar epithelial type II cells in primary culture. Physiol Rep. 2015;3(2) (Epub 2015/02/14).

46. Zhao L, Yee M, O'Reilly MA. Transdifferentiation of alveolar epithelial type II to type I cells is controlled by opposing TGF-beta and BMP signaling. Am J Physiol Lung Cell Mol Physiol. 2013;305(6):L409–18 (Epub 2013/07/09).

47. Mutze K, Vierkotten S, Milosevic J, Eickelberg O, Königshoff M. Enolase 1 (ENO1) and protein disulfide-isomerase associated 3 (PDIA3) regulate Wnt/beta-catenin-driven trans-differentiation of murine alveolar epithelial cells. Dis Models Mech. 2015;8(8):877–90 (Epub 2015/06/03).

48. Borok Z, Danto SI, Lubman RL, Cao Y, Williams MC, Crandall ED. Modulation of t1α expression with alveolar epithelial cell phenotype in vitro. Am J Physiol. 1998;275(1 Pt 1): L155–64 (Epub 1998/08/05).
49. Zhou B, Zhong Q, Minoo P, Li C, Ann DK, Frenkel B, et al. Foxp2 inhibits Nkx2.1-mediated transcription of SP-C via interactions with the Nkx2.1 homeodomain. Am J Respir Cell Mol Biol. 2008;38(6):750–8 (Epub 2008/02/02).
50. Pittet JF, Griffiths MJ, Geiser T, Kaminski N, Dalton SL, Huang X, et al. TGF-β is a critical mediator of acute lung injury. J Clin Investig. 2001;107(12):1537–44 (Epub 2001/06/20).
51. Gereke M, Autengruber A, Grobe L, Jeron A, Bruder D, Stegemann-Koniszewski S. Flow cytometric isolation of primary murine type II alveolar epithelial cells for functional and molecular studies. J Vis Exp JoVE. 2012;(70) (Epub 2013/01/05).
52. Lee JH, Kim J, Gludish D, Roach RR, Saunders AH, Barrios J, et al. Surfactant protein-C chromatin-bound green fluorescence protein reporter mice reveal heterogeneity of surfactant protein C-expressing lung cells. Am J Respir Cell Mol Biol. 2013;48(3):288–98 (Epub 2012/12/04).
53. Vanderbilt JN, Gonzalez RF, Allen L, Gillespie A, Leaffer D, Dean WB, et al. High-efficiency type II cell-enhanced green fluorescent protein expression facilitates cellular identification, tracking, and isolation. Am J Respir Cell Mol Biol. 2015;53(1):14–21 (Epub 2015/02/19).
54. Lo B, Hansen S, Evans K, Heath JK, Wright JR. Alveolar epithelial type II cells induce T cell tolerance to specific antigen. J Immunol. 2008;180(2):881–8 (Epub 2008/01/08).
55. Roper JM, Staversky RJ, Finkelstein JN, Keng PC, O'Reilly MA. Identification and isolation of mouse type II cells on the basis of intrinsic expression of enhanced green fluorescent protein. Am J Physiol Lung Cell Mol Physiol. 2003;285(3):L691–700 (Epub 2003/05/13).
56. Teisanu RM, Chen H, Matsumoto K, McQualter JL, Potts E, Foster WM, et al. Functional analysis of two distinct bronchiolar progenitors during lung injury and repair. Am J Respir Cell Mol Biol. 2011;44(6):794–803 (Epub 2010/07/27).
57. Messier EM, Mason RJ, Kosmider B. Efficient and rapid isolation and purification of mouse alveolar type II epithelial cells. Exp Lung Res. 2012;38(7):363–73 (Epub 2012/08/15).
58. Chapman HA, Li X, Alexander JP, Brumwell A, Lorizio W, Tan K, et al. Integrin α6β4 identifies an adult distal lung epithelial population with regenerative potential in mice. J Clin Investig. 2011;121(7):2855–62 (Epub 2011/06/28).
59. Van der Velden JL, Bertoncello I, McQualter JL. LysoTracker is a marker of differentiated alveolar type II cells. Respir Res. 2013;14:123 (Epub 2013/11/13).
60. Marconett CN, Zhou B, Rieger ME, Selamat SA, Dubourd M, Fang X, et al. Integrated transcriptomic and epigenomic analysis of primary human lung epithelial cell differentiation. PLoS Genetics. 2013;9(6):e1003513 (Epub 2013/07/03).
61. Daum N, Kuehn A, Hein S, Schaefer UF, Huwer H, Lehr CM. Isolation, cultivation, and application of human alveolar epithelial cells. Methods Mol Biol. 2012;806:31–42 Epub 2011/11/08.
62. Wang J, Wang S, Manzer R, McConville G, Mason RJ. Ozone induces oxidative stress in rat alveolar type II and type I-like cells. Free Radic Biol Med. 2006;40(11):1914–28 (Epub 2006/05/24).
63. Dobbs LG, Williams MC, Brandt AE. Changes in biochemical characteristics and pattern of lectin binding of alveolar type II cells with time in culture. Biochim Biophys Acta. 1985;846 (1):155–66 (Epub 1985/07/30).
64. Borok Z, Lubman RL, Danto SI, Zhang XL, Zabski SM, King LS, et al. Keratinocyte growth factor modulates alveolar epithelial cell phenotype in vitro: expression of aquaporin 5. Am J Respir Cell Mol Biol. 1998;18(4):554–61 (Epub 1998/05/02).
65. Fehrenbach H, Kasper M, Tschernig T, Pan T, Schuh D, Shannon JM, et al. Keratinocyte growth factor-induced hyperplasia of rat alveolar type II cells in vivo is resolved by differentiation into type I cells and by apoptosis. Eur Respir J. 1999;14(3):534–44 (Epub 1999/10/30).

66. Yano T, Mason RJ, Pan T, Deterding RR, Nielsen LD, Shannon JM. KGF regulates pulmonary epithelial proliferation and surfactant protein gene expression in adult rat lung. Am J Physiol Lung Cell Mol Physiol. 2000;279(6):L1146–58 (Epub 2000/11/15).

67. Isakson BE, Lubman RL, Seedorf GJ, Boitano S. Modulation of pulmonary alveolar type II cell phenotype and communication by extracellular matrix and KGF. Am J Physiol Cell Physiol. 2001;281(4):C1291–9 (Epub 2001/09/08).

68. Wang J, Edeen K, Manzer R, Chang Y, Wang S, Chen X, et al. Differentiated human alveolar epithelial cells and reversibility of their phenotype in vitro. Am J Respir Cell Mol Biol. 2007;36(6):661–8 (Epub 2007/01/27).

69. Gonzales LW, Guttentag SH, Wade KC, Postle AD, Ballard PL. Differentiation of human pulmonary type II cells in vitro by glucocorticoid plus cAMP. Am J Physiol Lung Cell Mol Physiol. 2002;283(5):L940–51 (Epub 2002/10/12).

70. Weng T, Poth JM, Karmouty-Quintana H, Garcia-Morales LJ, Melicoff E, Luo F, et al. Hypoxia-induced deoxycytidine kinase contributes to epithelial proliferation in pulmonary fibrosis. Am J Respir Crit Care Med. 2014;190(12):1402–12 (Epub 2014/10/31).

71. Tsuji T, Aoshiba K, Nagai A. Alveolar cell senescence in patients with pulmonary emphysema. Am J Respir Crit Care Med. 2006;174(8):886–93 (Epub 2006/08/05).

72. Tickner J, Fan LM, Du J, Meijles D, Li JM. Nox2-derived ROS in PPARgamma signaling and cell-cycle progression of lung alveolar epithelial cells. Free Radic Biol Med. 2011;51 (3):763–72 (Epub 2011/06/15).

73. Ochieng JK, Schilders K, Kool H, Boerema-De Munck A, Buscop-Van Kempen M, Gontan C, et al. Sox2 regulates the emergence of lung basal cells by directly activating the transcription of Trp63. Am J Respir Cell Mol Biol. 2014;51(2):311–22 (Epub 2014/03/29).

74. Falfan-Valencia R, Camarena A, Juarez A, Becerril C, Montano M, Cisneros J, et al. Major histocompatibility complex and alveolar epithelial apoptosis in idiopathic pulmonary fibrosis. Hum Genet. 2005;118(2):235–44 (Epub 2005/09/01).

75. Ballweg K, Mutze K, Königshoff M, Eickelberg O, Meiners S. Cigarette smoke extract affects mitochondrial function in alveolar epithelial cells. Am J Physiol Lung Cell Mol Physiol. 2014;307(11):L895–907 (Epub 2014/10/19).

76. Mercer PF, Woodcock HV, Eley JD, Plate M, Sulikowski MG, Durrenberger PF, et al. Exploration of a potent PI3 kinase/mTOR inhibitor as a novel anti-fibrotic agent in IPF. Thorax. 2016 (Epub 2016/04/23).

77. Pagano A, Pitteloud C, Reverdin C, Metrailler-Ruchonnet I, Donati Y. Barazzone Argiroffo C. Poly(ADP-ribose)polymerase activation mediates lung epithelial cell death in vitro but is not essential in hyperoxia-induced lung injury. Am J Respir Cell Mol Biol. 2005;33(6):555–64 (Epub 2005/09/10).

78. Tanjore H, Degryse AL, Crossno PF, Xu XC, McConaha ME, Jones BR, et al. beta-catenin in the alveolar epithelium protects from lung fibrosis after intratracheal bleomycin. Am J Respir Crit Care Med. 2013;187(6):630–9 (Epub 2013/01/12).

79. Drakopanagiotakis F, Xifteri A, Polychronopoulos V, Bouros D. Apoptosis in lung injury and fibrosis. Eur Respir J. 2008;32(6):1631–8 (Epub 2008/12/02).

80. Bartis D, Mise N, Mahida RY, Eickelberg O, Thickett DR. Epithelial-mesenchymal transition in lung development and disease: does it exist and is it important? Thorax. 2014;69 (8):760–5 (Epub 2013/12/18).

81. Moustakas A, Heldin CH. Mechanisms of TGFbeta-induced epithelial-mesenchymal transition. J Clin Med. 2016;5(7) (Epub 2016/07/02).

82. Nieto MA, Huang RY, Jackson RA, Thiery JP. Emt: 2016. Cell. 2016;166(1):21–45 (Epub 2016/07/02).

83. Willis BC, Liebler JM, Luby-Phelps K, Nicholson AG, Crandall ED, du Bois RM, et al. Induction of epithelial-mesenchymal transition in alveolar epithelial cells by transforming growth factor-β1: potential role in idiopathic pulmonary fibrosis. Am J Pathol. 2005;166 (5):1321–32 (Epub 2005/04/28).

84. Kasai H, Allen JT, Mason RM, Kamimura T, Zhang Z. TGF-β1 induces human alveolar epithelial to mesenchymal cell transition (EMT). Respir Res. 2005;6:56 (Epub 2005/06/11).

85. Holgate ST, Holloway J, Wilson S, Bucchieri F, Puddicombe S, Davies DE. Epithelial-mesenchymal communication in the pathogenesis of chronic asthma. Proc Am Thorac Soc. 2004;1(2):93–8 (Epub 2005/08/23).

86. Kim KK, Kugler MC, Wolters PJ, Robillard L, Galvez MG, Brumwell AN, et al. Alveolar epithelial cell mesenchymal transition develops in vivo during pulmonary fibrosis and is regulated by the extracellular matrix. Proc Natl Acad Sci USA. 2006;103(35):13180–5 (Epub 2006/08/23).

87. Tanjore H, Xu XC, Polosukhin VV, Degryse AL, Li B, Han W, et al. Contribution of epithelial-derived fibroblasts to bleomycin-induced lung fibrosis. Am J Respir Crit Care Med. 2009;180(7):657–65 (Epub 2009/06/27).

88. Adamson IY, Bowden DH. The type 2 cell as progenitor of alveolar epithelial regeneration. A cytodynamic study in mice after exposure to oxygen. Lab Investig J Tech Methods Pathol. 1974;30(1):35–42 (Epub 1974/01/01).

89. Evans MJ, Cabral LJ, Stephens RJ, Freeman G. Transformation of alveolar type 2 cells to type 1 cells following exposure to NO2. Exp Mol Pathol. 1975;22(1):142–50 (Epub 1975/02/01).

90. Treutlein B, Brownfield DG, Wu AR, Neff NF, Mantalas GL, Espinoza FH, et al. Reconstructing lineage hierarchies of the distal lung epithelium using single-cell RNA-seq. Nature. 2014;509(7500):371–5 (Epub 2014/04/18).

91. Vaughan AE, Brumwell AN, Xi Y, Gotts JE, Brownfield DG, Treutlein B, et al. Lineage-negative progenitors mobilize to regenerate lung epithelium after major injury. Nature. 2015;517(7536):621–5 (Epub 2014/12/24).

92. Dobbs LG. Isolation and culture of alveolar type II cells. Am J Physiol. 1990;258(4 Pt 1): L134–47 (Epub 1990/04/01).

93. Rishi AK, Joyce-Brady M, Fisher J, Dobbs LG, Floros J, VanderSpek J, et al. Cloning, characterization, and development expression of a rat lung alveolar type I cell gene in embryonic endodermal and neural derivatives. Dev Biol. 1995;167(1):294–306 (Epub 1995/01/01).

94. Williams MC, Cao Y, Hinds A, Rishi AK, Wetterwald A. T1 alpha protein is developmentally regulated and expressed by alveolar type I cells, choroid plexus, and ciliary epithelia of adult rats. Am J Respir Cell Mol Biol. 1996;14(6):577–85 (Epub 1996/06/01).

95. Dobbs LG, Williams MC, Gonzalez R. Monoclonal antibodies specific to apical surfaces of rat alveolar type I cells bind to surfaces of cultured, but not freshly isolated, type II cells. Biochim Biophys Acta. 1988;970(2):146–56 (Epub 1988/06/30).

96. Flozak AS, Lam AP, Russell S, Jain M, Peled ON, Sheppard KA, et al. β-catenin/T-cell factor signaling is activated during lung injury and promotes the survival and migration of alveolar epithelial cells. J Biol Chem. 2010;285(5):3157–67 (Epub 2009/11/26).

97. Nielsen S, King LS, Christensen BM, Agre P. Aquaporins in complex tissues. II. Subcellular distribution in respiratory and glandular tissues of rat. Am J Physiol. 1997;273(5 Pt 1): C1549–61 (Epub 1997/12/31).

98. Drab M, Verkade P, Elger M, Kasper M, Lohn M, Lauterbach B, et al. Loss of caveolae, vascular dysfunction, and pulmonary defects in caveolin-1 gene-disrupted mice. Science. 2001;293(5539):2449–52 (Epub 2001/08/11).

99. Razani B, Engelman JA, Wang XB, Schubert W, Zhang XL, Marks CB, et al. Caveolin-1 null mice are viable but show evidence of hyperproliferative and vascular abnormalities. J Biol Chem. 2001;276(41):38121–38 (Epub 2001/07/18).

100. Fuchs S, Hollins AJ, Laue M, Schaefer UF, Roemer K, Gumbleton M, et al. Differentiation of human alveolar epithelial cells in primary culture: morphological characterization and synthesis of caveolin-1 and surfactant protein-C. Cell Tissue Res. 2003;311(1):31–45 (Epub 2002/12/17).

101. Jain R, Barkauskas CE, Takeda N, Bowie EJ, Aghajanian H, Wang Q, et al. Plasticity of Hopx(+) type I alveolar cells to regenerate type II cells in the lung. Nature Commun. 2015;6:6727 (Epub 2015/04/14).

102. Shirasawa M, Fujiwara N, Hirabayashi S, Ohno H, Iida J, Makita K, et al. Receptor for advanced glycation end-products is a marker of type I lung alveolar cells. Genes Cells Devot Mol Cell Mech. 2004;9(2):165–74 (Epub 2004/03/11).

103. Wang Y, Huang C, Reddy Chintagari N, Bhaskaran M, Weng T, Guo Y, et al. miR-375 regulates rat alveolar epithelial cell trans-differentiation by inhibiting Wnt/β-catenin pathway. Nucleic Acids Res. 2013;41(6):3833–44 (Epub 2013/02/12).

104. Ghosh MC, Gorantla V, Makena PS, Luellen C, Sinclair SE, Schwingshackl A, et al. Insulin-like growth factor-I stimulates differentiation of ATII cells to ATI-like cells through activation of Wnt5a. Am J Physiol Lung Cell Mol Physiol. 2013;305(3):L222–8 (Epub 2013/05/28).

105. Bhaskaran M, Kolliputi N, Wang Y, Gou D, Chintagari NR, Liu L. Trans-differentiation of alveolar epithelial type II cells to type I cells involves autocrine signaling by transforming growth factor β1 through the Smad pathway. J Biol Chem. 2007;282(6):3968–76 (Epub 2006/12/13).

106. Gonzalez R, Yang YH, Griffin C, Allen L, Tigue Z, Dobbs L. Freshly isolated rat alveolar type I cells, type II cells, and cultured type II cells have distinct molecular phenotypes. Am J Physiol Lung Cell Mol Physiol. 2005;288(1):L179–89 (Epub 2004/09/28).

107. Lee JH, Bhang DH, Beede A, Huang TL, Stripp BR, Bloch KD, et al. Lung stem cell differentiation in mice directed by endothelial cells via a BMP4-NFATc1-thrombospondin-1 axis. Cell. 2014;156(3):440–55 (Epub 2014/02/04).

108. Clevers H. Modeling development and disease with organoids. Cell. 2016;165(7):1586–97 (Epub 2016/06/18).

109. Kleinman HK, Martin GR. Matrigel: basement membrane matrix with biological activity. Semin Cancer Biol. 2005;15(5):378–86 (Epub 2005/06/25).

Chapter 7
Flow Cytometric Evaluation of Acute Lung Injury and Repair

Jason R. Mock, Benjamin D. Singer and Franco R. D'Alessio

Abbreviations

AF	Autofluorescence
APC	Allophycocyanin
AT1	Type 1 alveolar epithelial cell
AT2	Type 2 alveolar epithelial cell
BAL	Bronchoalveolar lavage
CD	Cluster of differentiation
DNA	Deoxyribonucleic acid
ELISA	Enzyme-linked immunosorbent assay
FCS	Flow cytometry standard
FITC	Fluorescein isothiocyanate
FSC	Forward scatter
GFP	Green fluorescent protein
NADPH	Nicotinamide adenine dinucleotide phosphate
PE	Phycoerythrin
PMA	Phorbol myristate acetate
PMT	Photomultiplier tubes
SSC	Side scatter
SP-C	Surfactant protein C

J.R. Mock
Division of Pulmonary Diseases and Critical Care Medicine, University of North Carolina
School of Medicine, 130 Mason Farm Road CB#7020, Chapel Hill, NC 27599, USA
e-mail: jason_mock@med.unc.edu

B.D. Singer
Division of Pulmonary and Critical Care Medicine, Northwestern University Feinberg School
of Medicine, 240 E. Huron Street, McGaw M-300, Chicago, IL 60611, USA
e-mail: bsinger007@fsm.northwestern.edu

F.R. D'Alessio (✉)
Division of Pulmonary and Critical Care Medicine, Johns Hopkins Asthma and Allergy
Center, 5501 Hopkins Bayview Circle, Room 4B.51A, Baltimore, MD 21224, USA
e-mail: fdaless2@jhmi.edu

© Springer International Publishing AG 2017
L.M. Schnapp and C. Feghali-Bostwick (eds.), *Acute Lung Injury and Repair*,
Respiratory Medicine, DOI 10.1007/978-3-319-46527-2_7

Introduction

The lung is a complex organ that contains multiple cell types, including epithelial cells, endothelial cells, lymphatic cells, fibroblasts, pericytes, macrophages, and lymphocytes. In addition, we are recognizing that each of the cell populations are quite heterogeneous and contain distinct subpopulations. Determining the contribution of different cell types, and understanding expression profiles of discrete cell populations is critical to advance our understanding of many lung processes, including acute lung injury. The ability to measure multiple parameters of a single cell by flow cytometry provides a powerful technique for understanding cellular processes, and flow cytometry has become a valuable tool for studying cell biology including pulmonary research [1]. Through such methods as enzymatic and mechanical digestion of tissues, the increasing ability to measure greater numbers of fluorescence parameters in a single experiment, and the increase in commercially available fluorescently labeled antibodies and other fluorescent reagents have allowed the flow cytometer to become a common technique in the study of cells derived from solid organs [2–7]. Flow cytometry represents a potent technique utilized by lung researchers to uncover important mechanisms which could improve the understanding of pathology and disease processes in the lung. The purpose of this chapter is to familiarize the reader to some of the basics of flow cytometry, especially where this technology has been of particular benefit to the study of lung injury and repair.

Covering all the fundamentals of flow cytometry is outside the scope of this chapter, and there are excellent references and reviews which can introduce new users of flow cytometry to the nuts and bolts of fluidics, optical systems, and fluorescence along with providing detailed protocols for data acquisition and analysis (Table 7.1) [1, 7–9]. Flow cytometry is a unique approach to cellular investigation in that it can provide information on a single cell as part of a larger population. Flow cytometry detects cell size and their components (surface or intracellular) using fluorochromes attached to antibodies or chemical probes for specific cellular targets. Fluorochromes are molecules which absorb light of one wavelength and emit light at another wavelength. Over the last several decades there has been an increase in the number and availability of fluorochromes for study in flow cytometry. Newer fluorochromes (such as quantum dots) have very narrow emission peaks allowing for more parameters to be studied in a single experiment. Fluorochromes, when excited by a specific wavelength, will emit light which can then be separated out from other fluorochromes through a system of filters and mirrors before measurement by photomultiplier tubes (PMTs) or fiber array photo diodes (FAPDs). Simultaneous measurements of numerous parameters on each cell can be determined without the need for prior purification, which offers a method of analysis where information on each cell in the total population is stored in a database that can then be interrogated as part of specific population or

Table 7.1 Resources for further study of flow cytometry methods and applications

General

Practical Flow Cytometry, 4th Edition. Howard M. Shapiro. Wiley-Liss (2003)

Flow Cytometry: A Practical Approach, 3rd Edition. M.G. Ormerod. Oxford University Press (2000)

Cell Separation: Fundamentals, Analytical and Preparative Method. A. Kumar, I.Y. Galaev, and B. Mattiasson. Springer 2007

Garn H. *Specific aspects of flow cytometric analysis of cells from the lung.* Exp Toxicol Pathol. 2006 Jun;57 Suppl 2:21–4

Hawley TS, Herbert DJ, Eaker SS, Hawley RG. *Multiparameter flow cytometry of fluorescent protein reporters.* Methods Mol Biol. 2004;263:219–38

Preparing lung cells for flow cytometry

Martin J, White IN. *Preparation of rat lung cells for flow cytometry.* Methods Mol Biol. 1992;10:363–8

Gereke M, Autengruber A, Grobe L, Jeron A, Bruder D, Stegemann-Koniszewski S. *Flow cytometric isolation of primary murine type II alveolar epithelial cells for functional and molecular studies.* J Vis Exp. 2012 (70)

Jungblut M, Oeltze K, Zehnter I, Hasselmann D, Bosio A. *Standardized preparation of single-cell suspensions from mouse lung tissue using the gentleMACS Dissociator.* J Vis Exp. 2009 (29)

Kim CF, Jackson EL, Woolfenden AE, Lawrence S, Babar I, Vogel S, et al. *Identification of bronchioalveolar stem cells in normal lung and lung cancer.* Cell. 2005 Jun 17;121(6):823–35

Sauer KA, Scholtes P, Karwot R, Finotto S. *Isolation of CD4+ T cells from murine lungs: a method to analyze ongoing immune responses in the lung.* Nat Protoc. 2006;1(6):2870–5

Mouse myeloid immunophenotyping

Misharin et al. *Flow Cytometric Analysis of Macrophages and Dendritic Cells Subsets in the Mouse Lung.* Am J Respir Cell Mol Biol. 2013 Oct;49(4):503–10

Zaynagetdinov et al. *Identification of Myeloid Cell Subsets in Murine Lungs Using Flow Cytometry.* Am J Respir Cell Mol Biol. 2013 Aug;49(2): 180–9

Aggarwal et al. *Diverse Macrophage Populations Mediate Acute Lung Inflammation and Resolution.* Am J Physiol Lung Cell Mol Physiol. 2014 Apr 15;306 (8):L709–25

Mouse epithelial immunophenotyping

Bantikassegn et al. *Isolation of Epithelial, Endothelial, and Immune Cells from Lungs of Transgenic Mice with Oncogene-Induced Lung Adenocarcinomas.* Am J Respir Cell Mol Biol. 2015 Apr;52(4):409–17

Li et al. *Diversity of Epithelial Stem Cell Types in Adult Lung. Stem Cells International.* Volume 2015;728307

Mock et al. *Foxp3 regulatory T cells promote lung epithelial proliferation.* Mucosal Immunol. 2014 Nov;7(6):1440–51

Vaughan AE, Brumwell AN, Xi Y, Gotts JE, Brownfield DG, Treutlein B, et al. *Lineage-negative progenitors mobilize to regenerate lung epithelium after major injury.* Nature. 2015 Jan 29;517(7536):621–5

Barkauskas CE, Cronce MJ, Rackley CR et al. *Type 2 alveolar cells are stem cells in adult lung.* JCI 2013;Jul 1: 123(7): 3025–3036

(continued)

Table 7.1 (continued)

Human lung population identification
Fujino et al. *A novel method for isolating individual cellular components from the adult human distal lung*. Am J Respir Cell Mol Biol. 2012 Apr;46(4):422–30
Umino T, Skold CM, Pirruccello SJ, Spurzem JR, Rennard SI. *Two-color flow cytometric analysis of pulmonary alveolar macrophages from smokers*. Eur Respir J. 1999 Apr;13(4):894–9
Harbeck RJ. *Immunophenotyping of bronchoalveolar lavage lymphocytes*. Clin Diagn Lab Immunol. 1998 May;5(3):271–7
Maus U, Rosseau S, Seeger W, Lohmeyer J. *Separation of human alveolar macrophages by flow cytometry*. Am J Physiol. 1997 Mar;272(3 Pt 1):L566–71
Krombach F, Gerlach JT, Padovan C, Burges A, Behr J, Beinert T, et al. *Characterization and quantification of alveolar monocyte-like cells in human chronic inflammatory lung disease*. Eur Respir J. 1996 May;9(5):984–91
Whitehead BF, Stoehr C, Finkle C, Patterson G, Theodore J, Clayberger C, et al. *Analysis of bronchoalveolar lavage from human lung transplant recipients by flow cytometry*. Respir Med. 1995 Jan;89(1):27–34

Publishing flow cytometry data
Lee et al. *MIFlowCyt: The Minimum Information About a Flow Cytometry Experiment*. Cytometry Part A. 73A:926–30, 2008
Alvarez et al. *Publishing flow cytometry data*. Am J Physiol Lung Cell Mol Physiol 298: L127–130, 2010
Parks et al. *A new "Logicle" display method avoids deceptive effects of logarithmic scaling for low signals and compensated data*. Cytometry A 2006;69:542–51
Roederer et al. *Guidelines for the presentation of flow cytometric data*. Methods Cell Biol. 2004;75:241–56

group. Furthermore, a fundamental difference of flow cytometry compared to other traditional quantitative approaches (i.e., immunoblot and ELISA) is that the cells can be isolated (cell sorting) for further downstream applications based on expression of molecules specific to a certain cell population of interest. The two prerequisites required for each experiment are: (1) cells need to be in suspension and (2) cells should have as little nonspecific fluorescence (autofluorescence) as possible at emission wavelengths for the fluorochromes used in the experiment. One of the major drawbacks of flow cytometry is that single cells suspensions are required which necessitates disruption of the underlying tissue structure.

Obtaining Cell Suspensions

One of the most important considerations for flow cytometry of lung cells is how best to obtain single-cell populations for analysis. There are an estimated 40 cell types in the lung including mesenchymal lineages (vascular endothelial cells, lymphatic cells, pericytes, and fibrocytes), hematopoietic lineages (dendritic cells, lymphocytes, macrophages, and neutrophils) and epithelial lineages (neuroendocrine, basal, club, ciliated, goblet, type 1 and type 2 alveolar epithelial cells) along with several putative progenitor cells recently discovered [2, 3, 10, 11]. This diversity is further compounded by the multiple different compartments that make up the lung such as the bronchoalveolar space, vasculature, lymphatics, interstitium, and epithelium. These compartments can further be partitioned in respect to spatial dimension (i.e., proximal vs. distal) [12].

Obtaining cells for flow cytometry from certain lung compartments is easier than others. For example, cells from a bronchoalveolar lavage (BAL) consistent of mainly myeloid cells already in single-cell suspension. Cells can be obtained from this compartment by inserting a cannula via the airways and instilling a solution such as saline into the airspace and aspirating back to lavage the lung and obtain the cells located at the alveolar space. This compartment has been the most extensively studied compartment in both animal models of acute lung injury and human flow cytometry experiments due to the availability of obtaining cells for analysis [12].

Other areas in the lung such as the interstitium, vasculature, and epithelium must first be either enzymatically digested or mechanically dissociated to obtain cells in suspension [12–15]. In some instances either method may have similar yield of cell types [16]; however, with enzymatic digestion the protease(s) used may cleave proteins of interest affecting identification and analysis [12, 13, 17]. This is an important aspect that should be considered when initiating a flow cytometry study and should be evaluated for each molecule of interest. For example, enzymatic digestion with one protease such as Dispase could disrupt antibody specific recognition of a particular surface receptor compared to another protease such as collagenase (Fig. 7.1). Table 7.1 provides a list of references describing the numerous methodologies for isolating and identifying specific populations from the lung and its different compartments before, during, and after injury.

Fig. 7.1 Example histogram plot comparing epitope recognition of a surface cell receptor from lungs which have been digested with either collagenase (*red*) or dispase (*blue*)

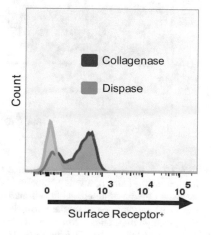

Fluorescence Acquisition

Signal intensity is directly related to the voltage applied to the PMT detector. For most applications the voltage is set to place the nonfluorescent cells (negative population) within the lower part of the measured scale. The intensities measured by the PMT are recorded and can be displayed in either a linear or logarithmic scale. The linear scale is generally used for depicting forward scatter (FSC, i.e., size), side scatter (SSC, i.e., granularity) or DNA content. A logarithmic scale is utilized for fluorescent marker applications given the wider order of magnitude with fluorescent signals [18].

There are several ways to present flow cytometric data. One of the more common methods is by displaying data for one parameter as a histogram in respect to measured fluorescence intensity (Fig. 7.2a). This graph displays the intensity of a signal (fluorescence) on the x-axis with the number of events (cells or count) on the y-axis, and can be used to obtain quantitative data about a specific marker. Two or more populations from different groups can be displayed by superimposing individual histograms assigned as different colors (Fig. 7.2a; red—whole lung single cell suspension versus blue—trachea single cell suspension only).

A second common method is by a dot plot to display information for two parameters. This type of presentation graphs the two parameters for each single cell and displays the data as a single dot (Fig. 7.2b; fluorescence intensity vs. SSC). Two parameter acquisition is often used to identify and measure subpopulations

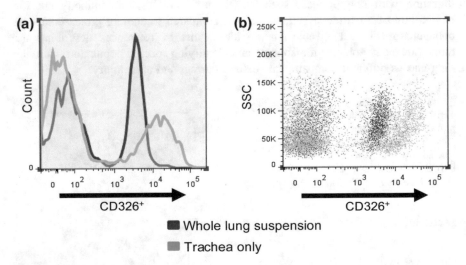

Fig. 7.2 a Example analysis comparing two different population samples (whole lung—*red*; trachea only—*blue*) in a one parameter histogram plot comparing APC-Cy7 fluorescence signal intensity (x-axis) of an epithelial cell marker, CD326 (EpCAM). The number of events or counts (i.e. cells) are represented on the y-axis. **b** Example analysis of a two parameter acquisition with a dot pot graph displaying information for two parameters with the same two single cell suspensions comparing CD326 APC-Cy7 fluorescence intensity (x-axis) to side scatter (granularity)

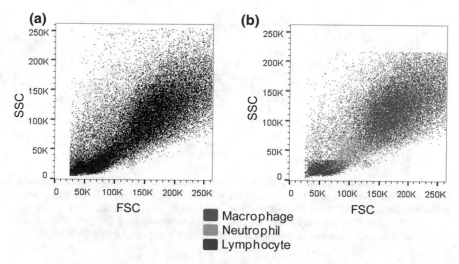

Fig. 7.3 Representative dot plot of cells from a mouse bronchoalveolar lavage in a two parameter acquisition (FSC vs. SSC). Based on comparing these two parameters, morphological differences in specific cell types can be seen. Color coded for macrophages (*pink*; CD11c), neutrophils (*green*; Ly6G) and lymphocytes (*red*; CD3)

from a larger population in the single-cell suspensions. These subgroups are often further evaluated in histogram plots for analyses. The FSC versus SSC dot plot is frequently the starting point for most flow cytometric data analysis. The FSC versus SSC dot plot can provide morphological data for cell samples and identify subpopulations such as lymphocytes, neutrophils, and macrophages such as in a mouse bronchoalveolar lavage sample (Fig. 7.3).

Areas of signal intensity can be identified and subdivided by selecting specific areas on the data plot (region gating) either in one parameter histograms or two parameter dot plots. The other setting to provide information on subpopulations is gating. A gate is assigned by the computer after a region is marked. A region can only include one or two parameters; however, a gate can encompass numerous regions, and can be used to select for a smaller specific population or subset within the sample passed through the cytometer.

Doublet Exclusion

One important step in data acquisition is to discriminate against events where two or more cells have been interrogated by the cytometer and measured as a single event. This can lead to misleading data. Evaluation for cell doublets (two cells attached to one another) is performed by measuring the cell's area versus either the cell's peak width or height and plotting both parameters against one another. This gating strategy allows for identification of a single spherical cellular subpopulation,

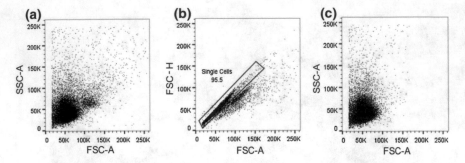

Fig. 7.4 **a** Representative dot plot of cells from mouse splenocytes in a two parameter acquisition (FSC vs. SSC). **b** Example gating strategy for determination of single cells identification by doublet exclusion by measuring FSC area vs. FSC height to discriminate against events where two or more cells have been interrogated by the cytometer simultaneously. **c** Dot plot of quadrangle from panel B in two parameter acquisition (FSC vs. SSC) identifying single cells

allowing for only apportioning just the single cells population to be further analyzed. An example of doublet exclusion is provided in Fig. 7.4 with the gating strategy demonstrated for identification of single cells by measuring FSC area vs. FSC height to discriminate against events where two or more cells have been interrogated by the cytometer simultaneously.

Compensation

Most fluorochromes after excitation can emit light over a range of wavelengths, and this spread can lead to signal overlap in data analysis when more than one fluorochrome is used. A flow cytometer can select out specific wavelengths before analysis by the PMT by passing the light emitted by the fluorochrome through a bandpass filter covering a specific wavelength range; however, even with these filters in place the PMT may register the overlap of undesired emission spectra from other fluorochromes. This overlap can result in the data being susceptible to incorrect assumptions [19]. Therefore, when more than one fluorochrome is used it is important to take into account the potential overlap of all the fluorochromes' emission spectra into the desired fluorochrome's spectra that will be measured by the PMT. Correcting or subtracting out this overlap between emission spectra must be performed for each experiment. One method is by performing single fluorochrome (color) staining of cells or synthetic beads and measuring overlap or spillover into the other PMT channels being used in the experiment. Using beads which can bind antibodies instead of cells is another method for compensation analysis and can avoid issues surrounding potentially low marker-density on a single-stained generic cell. A compensation sample will be needed for each fluorochrome used in an experiment (i.e., seven fluorochromes used necessitates seven individual tubes containing only one of the seven fluorochromes). Therefore one fluorochrome's (single-stained positive control) emission spectra can then be recorded by all the detectors in use for the experiment (primary detector and then the other peripheral detectors). Subtracting out the percentages of signal registered in the primary detector from the signal in the peripheral detector is termed compensation. Importantly, compensation values depend on the PMT voltages values for an experiment, which are set by the user, and any changes in voltages will negate current compensation settings and require them to be determined again. Most compensation algorithms also compare positive singly stained samples with a universal unstained negative cell population. This unstained sample may also assist when cells have background fluorescence (autofluorescence) and this can be identified and compensated for also by measuring fluorescence values of unlabeled (unstained) cells through the flow cytometry as a negative control.

Autofluorescence

Alveolar macrophages are the most numerous cells in BAL fluid of uninjured animals and humans. One characteristic relevant to flow cytometry of lung injury and repair is that this cell population can have a high level of autofluorescence (AF) [12]. AF is defined as natural emission of light from absorbed light by biological structures. Common AF molecules include: NADPH, flavin, collagen, lipofuscin, and metallo-proteins [12]. While AF can help identify a population, more often AF can complicate flow analysis. AF of alveolar macrophages occurs at an excitation wavelength of 488 nm which is a standard laser in cytometers, and can obfuscate signals from fluorescence dyes such as fluorescein isothiocyanate (FITC) or phycoerythrin (PE). Smoking can increase AF in alveolar macrophages [20]. AF of alveolar macrophages is lower at higher wavelengths used in flow cytometry, and fluorochromes such as allophycocyanin (APC) that are excited and emit light at higher wavelengths can assist in overcoming the complication of AF [12, 21]. Other methods include the use of tandem dyes or the use of quenching dyes (crystal violet or trypan blue) to reduce AF; however, the later requires the cells to be fixed and permeabilized before their application [12, 22, 23].

Fc Receptor Blockade

Some cells types express Fc receptors (CD16, CD32, CD64) such as macrophages and monocytes. Fluorochrome-conjugated antibodies can bind to both the specific antigen epitope and nonspecifically to Fc receptors. Blocking Fc receptors with an antibody specific for Fc receptors before application of the fluorochrome-conjugated antibodies can help negate this effect and increase antibody specificity. Fc receptor blockade is most useful when determining signal backgrounds with isotype fluorochrome-conjugated antibody controls so as to block nonspecific binding of the isotype antibody to a cell's Fc receptors [8]. Without blocking this potential inter-action there can be a falsely high estimation of background fluorescence to fluor-ochrome fluorescence signal. This application step is also useful if cells are prepared in protein-free buffers.

Building a Multicolor Flow Cytometry Panel

The expansion of novel fluorochromes makes building a multicolor flow cytometry panel challenging. Adequate panel design and antibody and instrument optimization are critical to obtain quality results. There are several principles to consider and include familiarizing with your instruments (e.g., lasers, PMT/filters, etc); using fluorochromes based on their relative brightness (e.g., choosing brighter dyes for lower abundant cell markers), minimizing spillovers and using appropriate biological and staining controls.

Given the potential for nonspecific staining when using multicolor flow cytometry, particularly for low abundant markers, the inclusion of Fluorescent minus One (FMO) should be considered. It represents a sample that contains all the fluorochromes in the panel except the one you are trying to measure (e.g., if a panel contains W, X, Y, and Z; the FMO for Z will only contain W, X, and Y). It is used to appropriately identify and gate cells for that specific marker measured.

Data Analysis

Flow cytometric data can be reported as cell-population data such as size and percentage (i.e., dot plot parameters) or may be quantitative based on fluorescent signal analysis (i.e., histograms of a fluorescent signal parameter). Estimating population size and determining the percentage of a population compared to the total cell population are common uses of flow cytometry. Of note, determining absolute numbers of cells is not a design of flow cytometry; however, there are methods to do so such as including fluorescent beads in the sample [24]. The histogram analysis can provide information on the percentage of a population in the region of interest along with quantitative data for the fluorescence emitted in the form of arithmetic or geometric means along with median values. Quantifying the fluorescence signal for a fluorochrome is proportional to the amount of fluor-ochrome bound to the cell; however, this measurement is dependent on the voltage setting which can be changed in each experiment. Choosing between arithmetic mean, geometric mean, or median values depends on the type of analysis [18, 25]. For log-amplified data using the geometric mean is more common, as it accounts for data distribution while arithmetic mean is used for data displayed on a linear scale. The median value of a population is often used, as the median is less influenced by skewed populations or outliers.

The flow cytometry standard (FCS) file format is the common file storage method implemented by most flow cytometer manufacturers and software applications [9]. This standardized format allows users to read files and examine data across many different cytometry and data analysis programs. The current file format, FSC 3.0, allows for handling files larger than 100 MB [9].

Cell Sorting

An important application of flow cytometry is the ability to sort highly purified cell populations from a heterogeneous mixture of cells for further downstream analyses. Typically, after a cell is interrogated by the cytometry lasers in the single-cell stream, it is collected in a waste container. In sorting, the cells or particles are identified and populations of interest are gated from identified regions, which can then be used to separate out (i.e., sort) cells from the fluid stream into collection tubes. An important consideration in sorting includes obtaining viable cells of interest after sorting and is best performed by keeping cells cooled to 4 °C. Another consideration is that sorting may damage the integrity of the cell membrane. Importantly, when sorting unfixed cells from potential biohazard samples precautions should be taken for safety from infectious materials. Sorters can produce aerosols, and it is recommended that instrument design, lab safety, and operator training be optimized. Many institutions, where sorting of potentially biohazardous material is done now carry out sorting in biosafety cabinets and negative pressure facilities. One important caveat is that when rare events or isolation of large populations are required it is often best to take advantage of bulk separation methods such as centrifugal separation or magnetic bead sorting to first enrich samples for the desired populations prior to cell sorting [26].

Transgenic Mice

The use of lung cell-specific transgenic mouse lines has facilitated progress in understanding processes in injury and repair [27, 28]. Numerous transgenic mouse strains have been constructed with lung-specific promoters such as *SFTPC* for AT2 cells, *Aqp5* for AT1 cells, *Scgb1a1* (also known as CCSP or CC10) for club cells, *Foxj1* for ciliated cells, and *Krt5* for basal cells [27]. Expression of GFP or other fluorescent reporters in these transgenic strains is a robust method for identification of populations and allowed for lineage tracing and downstream applications for 'omics' experiments. Sorting of cell populations from knockout or transgenic mice allows for the study of cell-specific roles of selected molecules [11, 29–31].

Applications in Lung Injury and Repair

Lung inflammation and the mechanisms involved in resolution after injury are important aspects to understanding disease processes in the lung. These processes involve interactions between different cell types during injury and repair. Flow cytometric methodologies permit the focused study of specific cell types throughout the course of injury and can assist in determining their specific roles as mediators of inflammation and repair. By uncovering the important cell-specific determinants of lung injury, researchers in the field will improve the understanding of lung disease pathophysiology and may allow for therapies to be discovered. An understanding of the fundamentals of flow cytometry above along with important particular lung-specific properties and techniques will equip investigators to efficiently utilize this technique and report flow cytometry data effectively [12].

Flow cytometric applications include: analysis of cell surface molecules to identify specific populations of cells in the lung (immunophenotyping), DNA proliferation and cell cycle analysis, cell viability, rates of cell death including differentiation between necrosis and apoptosis, protein expression, and protein phosphorylation status (Table 7.2) [12]. In lung injury and repair the most common use of flow cytometry is studying the immune system, both innate and adaptive, in regards to lung inflammation and repair [12].

Table 7.2 Flow cytometric applications

Cell surface
Phenotypic characterizations of surface proteins and their quantification
Immunophenotyping
Stem cell identification
Cell Sorting
Cell actions
Apoptosis and necrosis
Protein expression
Phagocytosis
Immune response
Cellular ion movement
Protein-protein interactions
Phosphorylation and kinase activity
Gene transcription
Cell kinetics
Cell proliferation
Cell cycle analysis
DNA content

Immunophenotyping

Identifying particular cell populations through detection of specific antigens (usually cell membrane proteins) from heterogeneous populations is termed immunophenotyping. Multicolor flow cytometry can be utilized to immunophenotype specific subpopulations in the lung using antibodies to identify specific antigens. Many of these antigens or markers are part of the cluster of differentiation (CD) system used to classify cell surface molecules [32]. Some of the more common surface markers can delineate endothelial (CD31), epithelial (CD326), and hematopoietic (CD45) lineages and have been reported throughout the lung injury literature [2, 3, 31, 33–36]. Further delineation of these subsets is possible, and detailed identification of specific populations is an active area of research in lung injury and repair [3, 34–36].

For example, identification of the myeloid cell populations in the lung is a common application of flow cytometry in the study of lung injury, and recently several papers have illustrated systematic approaches for identification of specific immune cell populations in the mouse lung during the course of injury and resolution (Table 7.1) [35–37]. These arrangements of antibodies and gating schemes used to identify specific populations of immune cells provide a useful tool to study the role of resident and recruited immune cell subsets in models of acute lung injury and inflammation. As more cell-specific markers are identified and populations confirmed by complementary methods, we should have improved insight into pulmonary immune responses.

Determining the role of epithelial populations in lung repair is another area of study, and immunophenotyping the epithelial populations involved by flow cytometry provides a methodology to better understand the role of the epithelial populations in lung repair [2–6, 33, 38]. The mechanisms underlying the reparative effects on lung epithelium regeneration are complex and involve progenitor populations, signaling pathways, and interaction with the extracellular matrix and immune cells [39]. The pan-epithelial markers CD326 and E-cadherin have been useful in identifying epithelial populations [40–42]. Numerous groups have used MHC class II molecules to identify type 2 alveolar epithelial cells (AT2) cells which have been previously described to be constitutively expressed on AT2 cells [33, 43–46]. As more cell-specific markers for epithelial populations are identified further delineation might be made available.

Epithelial progenitor populations have been identified through study of lung injury and reparative models with the aid of flow cytometry [2, 5, 11, 47–52]. Currently, there is intense interest in the role of progenitor populations in lung regeneration. The paradigm for repair of the alveolar epithelium after injury has been that type 1 alveolar epithelial cells (AT1) are susceptible to damage and more damage-resistant AT2 cells migrate to sites of injury and undergo hyperplasia and proliferation [51]. AT2 cells can then undergo differentiation to AT1 cells to reform an intact functional alveolar epithelial barrier [53, 54]. Several studies have questioned the AT2 progenitor paradigm as the sole progenitor of the alveolar epithelium and have established that several epithelial progenitor populations may also play a role in restoring an intact lung epithelium after injury [2, 5, 11, 31, 47–52]. Supporting the idea that other epithelial cell types are significant in repair, a study demonstrated through construction of an inducible surfactant protein C (SP-C) Cre reporter mouse that a subset of alveolar cells not expressing SP-C appeared to be important in repair after bleomycin injury [11]. Flow cytometric applications coupled with *in vivo* genetic lineage tracing studies will be helpful in determining the exact roles these progenitor populations play in repair [11, 31, 55]. The progenitor populations described have been characterized in mice and further work is required to determine if they are present and significant in human lung repair. Flow cytometry will likely be an important technique to confirm their presence and function in human lungs.

Cell Proliferation Methods

DNA analysis after immunophenotyping is a common flow cytometry application [8]. DNA content in the cell can be measured with fluorescent dyes that bind to DNA and the laser available on the cytometer can determine which dyes are suitable for use. One widely used dye is propidium iodide (PI); however, this dye is not DNA specific and can bind double-stranded RNA [8]. DAPI is another dye that works off of an ultraviolet or violet laser, but DAPI use requires that cells undergo permeabilization first. Hoechst 33342 is a dye that permits DNA content determination in viable cells without permeabilization. For optimal measurements with these dyes, preliminary experiments often need to be performed to determine the concentration and incubation times for optimal staining intensity [8]. Another method to determine proliferating cells is through intracellular staining for nuclear proteins associated with cellular proliferation such as ki-67, which is expressed in G_1, S, G_2 and M phases [56]. Another method is the dye dilution method where a dye is attached to a cell and as the cell divides the label is distributed between daughter cells and thus the fluorescence decreases. The number of cell divisions can be determined by following the dilution of the fluorescent label as the cells divide. Several compounds have been used for this application and include carboxyfluorescein diacetate, scuccinimidyl ester (CFSE), and PHK26 [8].

Investigators can determine changes in proliferation within different cell populations using these schemes. There are many other methods available and the resources listed in Table 7.1 provide further information on flow cytometry cell proliferation and cell cycle applications.

Cell Viability Analysis

There are various flow cytometric applications to identify and quantify viable cells in a sample. Determination can be important for a particular experiment, and also may be necessary to exclude dead cells from further downstream analysis. Dead cells can generate artifacts through nonspecific binding of antibodies or fluorescence probes. One method is dye exclusion such as with propidium iodide (PI), which binds to double-stranded DNA but is membrane-impermeable [8]. Another methodology relies on interaction of a fluorescent dye with specific molecules (amines) which will bind in low amounts to the surface of live cells but can penetrate the membrane in dead cells allowing for higher binding and an increase in fluorescent intensity [8]. Identifying cell viability and the protocols for doing so should be performed before fixation.

Cell Death

Annexin V binding is a common technique to detect cells undergoing apoptosis by flow cytometry. Annexin V binds phosphatidylserine, which under normal cell conditions resides on the inner plasma membrane but is externalized to the outer plasma membrane on apoptotic cells [57]. Proteins involved in apoptosis can be measured by flow cytometry if antibodies are available. Caspases are one family of apoptosis cascade proteins and their activity can be assessed using fluorescent substrates. Other methods are also available and include changes in mitochondrial membrane potential, DNA degradation, and the TUNEL assay that can all be utilized to study cell death by flow cytometry [8]. The resources listed in Table 7.1 provide further information on applications determining rates of cell death with flow cytometry such as applying these techniques to quantitating neutrophil apoptosis or efferocytosis.

Intracellular Staining Techniques

For identification and measurement of intracellular proteins, cells must first be fixed to ensure stability of antigens of interest. The next step requires that the cells undergo permeabilization prior to staining with the antibody-fluorochrome reagents. Importantly, antibody dilutions should be prepared in the permeabilization buffer to ensure the cells remain permeable. There are numerous procedures for staining intracellular antigens and the fixative and permeabilization steps often need to be optimized for each antigen as some fixatives and/or fixation time can adversely affect antigen recognition or fluorochromes (particularly conjugates like APC-Cy7 and fluorescent proteins like GFP) [8, 58].

For measurement of secreted proteins, compounds which inhibit protein secretion are used such as Brefeldin A [59, 60]. Brefeldin A is a fungal product that inhibits protein transport from the endoplasmic reticulum to the Golgi apparatus. Adding Brefeldin A to cultured cells a few hours before staining prevents proteins being released from the cell and enhances the resulting fluorescent signal. Additionally other compounds which stimulate secretory protein production such as ionomycin or phorbol myristate acetate (PMA) can be used to enhance signal and measure protein products from cells.

Measuring phosphorylation events by flow cytometry can provide insight into kinase signaling pathways, and flow cytometry can allow for multiple signals to be analyzed simultaneously [58]. Methods for optimal fixation and permeabilization have been studied and correlate with other methods such as immunoblotting. Similar to staining for intracellular antigens, the fixative and permeabilization steps often need to be optimized for each phosphoprotein of interest [58].

Human Flow Cytometry

BAL fluid and peripheral blood are the most commonly analyzed compartments in flow cytometry studies of human lung disease. Lung cancer samples post-surgery have also been used to study cancer cells but have also been a resource for evaluation of cellular components of the distal lung [3]. For the last several decades, analysis and immunophenotyping of cells from the BAL fluid from different patient populations have been performed (Table 7.1) [3, 20, 61–64]. As a better understanding of the inflammatory process and cellular determinants of resolution in mouse models of acute lung injury and repair are discovered, information obtained from animal models can be translated and expanded to human disease processes. Biohazard considerations should be employed when working with human samples. When sorting unfixed cells from potential biohazard samples precautions should be taken for safety from infectious materials, as sorters can produce infectious aerosols. It is recommended that instrument design, lab safety, and operator training be optimized. The resources listed in Table 7.1 provide further information on applications for analysis of BAL fluid samples along with methods for isolating individual cellular components form the adult distal lung.

Publishing Flow Data

As with most technologies, multiple methodologies exist for presenting data. In flow cytometry, these varying methods can result in questions regarding reproducibility which is further compounded by the lack of standardized methods for data presentation and publication [25]. This has further been complicated by the ability to analyze up to 20 different parameters for a single cell: multicolor flow analysis [65]. There are many references discussing guidelines for publishing flow cytometric data [25, 66, 67], and many journals have specific guidelines describing the requirements for flow cytometry data publication. Effectively reporting data allows for optimal interpretation and reproducibility, which is paramount in publishing flow cytometry results.

Several main points should be reported for flow cytometric data and analyses. First, a detailed description of both the experimental design and the preparation of single cell suspensions are important to help to ensure reproducibility. Authors should include detailed methods reporting: (1) enzymatic digestion or mechanical dissociation for obtaining single cells from tissue, (2) lysis of red blood cells, (3) cell filtration, (4) cell fixation and permeabilization, and (5) descriptions of the number or independent experiments along with number of samples in each experiment. Incorporating this information into a publication will provide a reader with the necessary methods to understand and potentially reproduce the data. Including the reagents used such as the antibodies, their conjugated fluorochromes, and information on vendor and catalog number are necessary. The manufacture and model of the flow cytometer used for the acquisition of data along with the laser configuration and filters used are notable [25]. The software program used during instrument acquisition along with the software used for analysis should be reported along with methods for fluorescence compensation.

For data analysis and presentation, the gating schemes used to define these populations should be outlined and include light scatter, live–dead discrimination, single cell (doublet exclusion), and fluorescent detecting gates. For fluorescent gates, information should be reported as to how comparisons made with the use of controls such as unstained controls, isotype controls, fluorescence-minus-one controls, or biologic controls [25].

Authors should report the statistical analysis used to determine significance and whether the analysis represents either percentage of cells for a specific gate or if fluorescence intensity was utilized [25]. Importantly if fluorescence intensity is utilized for data analysis, then reporting the method of instrument calibration to adjust or detect any changes and exclude potential changes in laser intensity over time between experiments should be included [25].

When presenting flow cytometric data in manuscripts, it is important to include actual cytometric data plots (versus bar graphs or tables) to accurately display the data and provide the information necessary for adequate interpretation [25]. This should be reported either within the manuscript figures or within supplemental data. The following references provided in Table 7.1 provide suggestions on how to display and report flow cytometry data. Overall, providing clear, detailed experimental setup along with information on instrument acquisition and data analysis is central to publishing cytometry data. While not required currently, one wonders if journals will turn to similar methods of data reporting and inclusion as has been done with other large scale data such as microarray and genome-wide sequencing data. In the future, journals could require authors to include raw FCS files with their supplemental data—providing such data may allow for better transparency of flow cytometry analysis and its interpretation.

Conclusion

Flow cytometry provides a powerful technique for understanding cellular processes in the lung and has become a popular methodology to interrogate processes important in injury and repair. Flow cytometric methods for identification of specific populations often build on the previous literature and reporting data effectively to provide for clarity and reproducibility is paramount. As more ways to identify and classify cells by cytometry are published, further delineation will be available in this rapidly progressing field. The provided resources can provide further information and one of the better approaches is to identify similar methodologies in the literature in areas of related research to best determine and optimize the protocols for your experimental analyses (Table 7.1). Also, flow cytometry core facilities and core facility operators can provide expertise regarding flow applications and methodologies. Becoming familiar with the essentials of flow cytometry and the methods and applications relevant to the study of lung injury and repair will help investigators better understand the literature and this method's potential for lung biology discovery.

We wish you success in your flow endeavors!

– Jason Mock, Benjamin Singer, and Franco D'Alessio.

References

1. Baumgarth N, Roederer M. A practical approach to multicolor flow cytometry for immunophenotyping. J Immunol Methods. 2000;243(1–2):77–97.
2. Kim CF, Jackson EL, Woolfenden AE, Lawrence S, Babar I, Vogel S, et al. Identification of bronchioalveolar stem cells in normal lung and lung cancer. Cell. 2005;121(6):823–35. PubMed PMID: 15960971 (Epub 2005/06/18. eng).
3. Fujino N, Kubo H, Ota C, Suzuki T, Suzuki S, Yamada M, et al. A novel method for isolating individual cellular components from the adult human distal lung. Am J Respir Cell Mol Biol. 2012;46(4):422–30. PubMed PMID: 22033268 (Epub 2011/10/29. eng).
4. Giangreco A, Shen H, Reynolds SD, Stripp BR. Molecular phenotype of airway side population cells. Am J Physiol Lung Cell Mol Physiol. 2004;286(4):L624–30.
5. Teisanu RM, Chen H, Matsumoto K, McQualter JL, Potts E, Foster WM, et al. Functional analysis of two distinct bronchiolar progenitors during lung injury and repair. Am J Respir Cell Mol Biol. 2011;44(6):794–803. PubMed PMID: 20656948. Pubmed Central PMCID: 3135841 (Epub 2010/07/27. eng).
6. Yamamoto K, Ferrari JD, Cao Y, Ramirez MI, Jones MR, Quinton LJ, et al. Type I alveolar epithelial cells mount innate immune responses during pneumococcal pneumonia. J Immunol. 2012;189(5):2450–9. PubMed PMID: 22844121. Pubmed Central PMCID: 3424336 (Epub 2012/07/31. eng).
7. Hawley TS, Herbert DJ, Eaker SS, Hawley RG. Multiparameter flow cytometry of fluorescent protein reporters. Methods Mol Biol. 2004;263:219–38.
8. Ormerod MG. Flow Cytometry—A basic introduction. 3rd ed. 2000.
9. Shapiro HM. Practical Flow Cytometry. 4th ed: Wiley-Liss; 2003.

10. Li F, He J, Wei J, Cho WC, Liu X. Diversity of epithelial stem cell types in adult lung. Stem Cells Int. 2015;2015:728307. PubMed PMID: 25810726. Pubmed Central PMCID: 4354973.

11. Chapman HA, Li X, Alexander JP, Brumwell A, Lorizio W, Tan K, et al. Integrin $\alpha6\beta4$ identifies an adult distal lung epithelial population with regenerative potential in mice. J Clin Invest. 2011;121(7):2855–62. PubMed PMID: 21701069 (Epub 2011/06/28. eng).

12. Garn H. Specific aspects of flow cytometric analysis of cells from the lung. Exp Toxicol Pathol. 2006;57(Suppl 2):21–4.

13. Martin J, White IN. Preparation of rat lung cells for flow cytometry. Methods Mol Biol. 1992;10:363–8.

14. Jungblut M, Oeltze K, Zehnter I, Hasselmann D, Bosio A. Standardized preparation of single-cell suspensions from mouse lung tissue using the gentleMACS Dissociator. J Vis Exp. 2009 (29). PubMed PMID: 19574953. Pubmed Central PMCID: 2798855.

15. Sauer KA, Scholtes P, Karwot R, Finotto S. Isolation of CD4+ T cells from murine lungs: a method to analyze ongoing immune responses in the lung. Nat Protoc. 2006;1(6):2870–5.

16. Fliegert FG, Tschernig T, Pabst R. Comparison of lymphocyte subsets, monocytes, and NK cells in three different lung compartments and peripheral blood in the rat. Exp Lung Res. 1996;22(6):677–90. PubMed PMID: 8979050.

17. Gereke M, Autengruber A, Grobe L, Jeron A, Bruder D, Stegemann-Koniszewski S. Flow cytometric isolation of primary murine type II alveolar epithelial cells for functional and molecular studies. J Vis Exp. 2012 (70). PubMed PMID: 23287741. Pubmed Central PMCID: 3576420.

18. Parks DR, Roederer M, Moore WA. A new "Logicle" display method avoids deceptive effects of logarithmic scaling for low signals and compensated data. Cytometry Part A J Int Soc Anal Cytol. 2006;69(6):541–51.

19. Bayer J, Grunwald D, Lambert C, Mayol JF, Maynadie M. Thematic workshop on fluorescence compensation settings in multicolor flow cytometry. Cytometry Part B Clin Cytometry. 2007;72(1):8–13.

20. Umino T, Skold CM, Pirruccello SJ, Spurzem JR, Rennard SI. Two-colour flow-cytometric analysis of pulmonary alveolar macrophages from smokers. Eur Respir J. 1999;13(4):894–9.

21. Fuchs HJ, McDowell J, Shellito JE. Use of allophycocyanin allows quantitative description by flow cytometry of alveolar macrophage surface antigens present in low numbers of cells. Am Rev Respir Dis. 1988;138(5):1124–8.

22. Hallden G, Skold CM, Eklund A, Forslid J, Hed J. Quenching of intracellular autofluorescence in alveolar macrophages permits analysis of fluorochrome labelled surface antigens by flow cytofluorometry. J Immunol Methods. 1991;142(2):207–14.

23. Viksman MY, Liu MC, Schleimer RP, Bochner BS. Application of a flow cytometric method using autofluorescence and a tandem fluorescent dye to analyze human alveolar macrophage surface markers. J Immunol Methods. 1994;172(1):17–24.

24. Nicholson JK, Stein D, Mui T, Mack R, Hubbard M, Denny T. Evaluation of a method for counting absolute numbers of cells with a flow cytometer. Clin Diagn Lab Immunol. 1997;4 (3):309–13. PubMed PMID: 9144369. Pubmed Central PMCID: 170524.

25. Alvarez DF, Helm K, Degregori J, Roederer M, Majka S. Publishing flow cytometry data. Am J Physiol Lung Cell Mol Physiol. 2010;298(2):L127–30. PubMed PMID: 19915158. Pubmed Central PMCID: 2822558.

26. Ibrahim SF, van den Engh G. Flow cytometry and cell sorting. Adv Biochem Eng Biotechnol. 2007;106:19–39.

27. Rawlins EL, Perl AK. The a"MAZE"ing world of lung-specific transgenic mice. Am J Respir Cell Mol Biol. 2012;46(3):269–82. PubMed PMID: 22180870. Pubmed Central PMCID: 3785140.

28. Baron RM, Choi AJ, Owen CA, Choi AM. Genetically manipulated mouse models of lung disease: potential and pitfalls. Am J Physiol Lung Cell Mol Physiol. 2012;302(6):L485–97 (PubMed PMID: 22198907. Pubmed Central PMCID: 4074003).

29. Fehrenbach ML, Cao G, Williams JT, Finklestein JM, Delisser HM. Isolation of murine lung endothelial cells. Am J Physiol Lung Cell Mol Physiol. 2009;296(6):L1096–103 (PubMed PMID: 19304908. Pubmed Central PMCID: 2692810).
30. Barkauskas CE. Type 2 alveolar cells are stem cells in adult lung. J Clin Invest. 2013.
31. Vaughan AE, Brumwell AN, Xi Y, Gotts JE, Brownfield DG, Treutlein B, et al. Lineage-negative progenitors mobilize to regenerate lung epithelium after major injury. Nature. 2015;517(7536):621–5 (PubMed PMID: 25533958. Pubmed Central PMCID: 4312207).
32. Chan JK, Ng CS, Hui PK. A simple guide to the terminology and application of leucocyte monoclonal antibodies. Histopathology. 1988;12(5):461–80.
33. Mock JR, Garibaldi BT, Aggarwal NR, Jenkins J, Limjunyawong N, Singer BD, et al. Foxp3 regulatory T cells promote lung epithelial proliferation. Mucosal Immunol. 2014. PubMed PMID: 24850425 (Epub 2014/05/23. Eng).
34. Bantikassegn A, Song X, Politi K. Isolation of epithelial, endothelial, and immune cells from lungs of transgenic mice with oncogene-induced lung adenocarcinomas. Am J Respir Cell Mol Biol. 2015;52(4):409–17.
35. Misharin AV, Morales-Nebreda L, Mutlu GM, Budinger GR, Perlman H. Flow cytometric analysis of macrophages and dendritic cell subsets in the mouse lung. Am J Respir Cell Mol Biol. 2013;49(4):503–10 (PubMed PMID: 23672262. Pubmed Central PMCID: 3824047).
36. Zaynagetdinov R, Sherrill TP, Kendall PL, Segal BH, Weller KP, Tighe RM, et al. Identification of myeloid cell subsets in murine lungs using flow cytometry. Am J Respir Cell Mol Biol. 2013;49(2):180–9. PubMed PMID: 23492192. Pubmed Central PMCID: 3824033.
37. Aggarwal NR, King LS, D'Alessio FR. Diverse macrophage populations mediate acute lung inflammation and resolution. Am J Physiol Lung Cell Mol Physiol. 2014;306(8):L709–25. PubMed PMID: 24508730. Pubmed Central PMCID: 3989724.
38. Lee JH, Kim J, Gludish D, Roach RR, Saunders AH, Barrios J, et al. SPC H2B-GFP mice reveal heterogeneity of surfactant protein C-expressing lung cells. Am J Respir Cell Mol Biol. 2012. PubMed PMID: 23204392 (Epub 2012/12/04. Eng).
39. Rock J, Konigshoff M. Endogenous lung regeneration: potential and limitations. Am J Respir Crit Care Med. 2012;186(12):1213–9. PubMed PMID: 22997206 (Epub 2012/09/22. eng).
40. Kauffman SL. Alterations in cell proliferation in mouse lung following urethane exposure. 3. Effects of chronic exposure on type 2 alveolar epithelial cell. Am J Pathol. 1972;68(2):317–26. PubMed PMID: 5049428. Pubmed Central PMCID: 2032677 (Epub 1972/08/01. eng).
41. Thaete LG, Beer DG, Malkinson AM. Genetic variation in the proliferation of murine pulmonary type II cells: basal rates and alterations following urethan treatment. Cancer Res. 1986;46(10):5335–8. PubMed PMID: 3756882 (Epub 1986/10/01. eng).
42. Evans MJ, Dekker NP, Cabral-Anderson LJ, Freeman G. Quantitation of damage to the alveolar epithelium by means of type 2 cell proliferation. Am Rev Respir Dis. 1978;118 (4):787–90. PubMed PMID: 707897 (Epub 1978/10/01. eng).
43. Lo B, Hansen S, Evans K, Heath JK, Wright JR. Alveolar epithelial type II cells induce T cell tolerance to specific antigen. J Immunol. 2008;180(2):881–8. PubMed PMID: 18178827 (Epub 2008/01/08. eng).
44. Cunningham AC, Milne DS, Wilkes J, Dark JH, Tetley TD, Kirby JA. Constitutive expression of MHC and adhesion molecules by alveolar epithelial cells (type II pneumocytes) isolated from human lung and comparison with immunocytochemical findings. J Cell Sci. 1994;107 (Pt 2):443–9. PubMed PMID: 8207072 (Epub 1994/02/01. eng).
45. Debbabi H, Ghosh S, Kamath AB, Alt J, Demello DE, Dunsmore S, et al. Primary type II alveolar epithelial cells present microbial antigens to antigen-specific CD4+ T cells. Am J Physiol Lung Cell Mol Physiol. 2005;289(2):L274–9. PubMed PMID: 15833765 (Epub 2005/04/19. eng).
46. Marsh LM, Cakarova L, Kwapiszewska G, von Wulffen W, Herold S, Seeger W, et al. Surface expression of CD74 by type II alveolar epithelial cells: a potential mechanism for macrophage migration inhibitory factor-induced epithelial repair. Am J Physiol Lung Cell Mol Physiol. 2009;296(3):L442–52. PubMed PMID: 19136583 (Epub 2009/01/13. eng).

47. Ding BS, Nolan DJ, Guo P, Babazadeh AO, Cao Z, Rosenwaks Z, et al. Endothelial-derived angiocrine signals induce and sustain regenerative lung alveolarization. Cell. 2011;147 (3):539–53. PubMed PMID: 22036563 (Epub 2011/11/01. eng).
48. Reynolds SD, Giangreco A, Power JH, Stripp BR. Neuroepithelial bodies of pulmonary airways serve as a reservoir of progenitor cells capable of epithelial regeneration. Am J Pathol. 2000;156(1):269–78. PubMed PMID: 10623675. Pubmed Central PMCID: 1868636 (Epub 2000/01/07. eng).
49. Rock JR, Randell SH, Hogan BL. Airway basal stem cells: a perspective on their roles in epithelial homeostasis and remodeling. Dis Model Mech. 2010;3(9–10):545–56. PubMed PMID: 20699479. Pubmed Central PMCID: 2931533 (Epub 2010/08/12. eng).
50. Kumar PA, Hu Y, Yamamoto Y, Hoe NB, Wei TS, Mu D, et al. Distal airway stem cells yield alveoli in vitro and during lung regeneration following H1N1 influenza infection. Cell. 2011;147(3):525–38. PubMed PMID: 22036562. Epub 2011/11/01. eng.
51. Evans MJ, Cabral LJ, Stephens RJ, Freeman G. Transformation of alveolar type 2 cells to type 1 cells following exposure to NO2. Exp Mol Pathol. 1975;22(1):142–50. PubMed PMID: 163758 (Epub 1975/02/01. eng).
52. Kajstura J, Rota M, Hall SR, Hosoda T, D'Amario D, Sanada F, et al. Evidence for human lung stem cells. N Engl J Med. 2011;364(19):1795–806. PubMed PMID: 21561345. Pubmed Central PMCID: 3197695 (Epub 2011/05/13. eng).
53. Fehrenbach H. Alveolar epithelial type II cell: defender of the alveolus revisited. Respir Res. 2001;2(1):33–46. PubMed PMID: 11686863. Pubmed Central PMCID: 59567 (Epub 2001/11/01. eng).
54. Adamson IY, Bowden DH. Derivation of type 1 epithelium from type 2 cells in the developing rat lung. Lab Invest. 1975;32(6):736–45. PubMed PMID: 1171339 (Epub 1975/06/01. eng).
55. Rock JR, Hogan BL. Epithelial progenitor cells in lung development, maintenance, repair, and disease. Annu Rev Cell Dev Biol. 2011;27:493–512. PubMed PMID: 21639799 (Epub 2011/06/07. eng).
56. Danova M, Riccardi A, Mazzini G. Cell cycle-related proteins and flow cytometry. Haematologica. 1990;75(3):252–64. PubMed PMID: 2146199 (Epub 1990/05/01. eng).
57. Henry CM, Hollville E, Martin SJ. Measuring apoptosis by microscopy and flow cytometry. Methods. 2013;61(2):90–7.
58. Krutzik PO, Nolan GP. Intracellular phospho-protein staining techniques for flow cytometry: monitoring single cell signaling events. Cytometry Part A J Int Soc Anal Cytol. 2003;55 (2):61–70.
59. Vicetti Miguel RD, Maryak SA, Cherpes TL. Brefeldin A, but not monensin, enables flow cytometric detection of interleukin-4 within peripheral T cells responding to ex vivo stimulation with Chlamydia trachomatis. J Immunol Methods. 2012;384(1–2):191–5. PubMed PMID: 22850275. Pubmed Central PMCID: 3444442.
60. Schuerwegh AJ, Stevens WJ, Bridts CH, De Clerck LS. Evaluation of monensin and brefeldin A for flow cytometric determination of interleukin-1 beta, interleukin-6, and tumor necrosis factor-alpha in monocytes. Cytometry. 2001;46(3):172–6.
61. Whitehead BF, Stoehr C, Finkle C, Patterson G, Theodore J, Clayberger C, et al. Analysis of bronchoalveolar lavage from human lung transplant recipients by flow cytometry. Respir Med. 1995;89(1):27–34.
62. Harbeck RJ. Immunophenotyping of bronchoalveolar lavage lymphocytes. Clin Diagn Lab Immunol. 1998;5(3):271–7. PubMed PMID: 9605975. Pubmed Central PMCID: 104508.
63. Maus U, Rosseau S, Seeger W, Lohmeyer J. Separation of human alveolar macrophages by flow cytometry. Am J Physiol. 1997;272(3 Pt 1):L566–71.
64. Krombach F, Gerlach JT, Padovan C, Burges A, Behr J, Beinert T, et al. Characterization and quantification of alveolar monocyte-like cells in human chronic inflammatory lung disease. Eur Respir J. 1996;9(5):984–91.

65. Chattopadhyay PK, Price DA, Harper TF, Betts MR, Yu J, Gostick E, et al. Quantum dot semiconductor nanocrystals for immunophenotyping by polychromatic flow cytometry. Nat Med. 2006;12(8):972–7.
66. Lee JA, Spidlen J, Boyce K, Cai J, Crosbie N, Dalphin M, et al. MIFlowCyt: the minimum information about a Flow Cytometry Experiment. Cytometry Part A: J Int Soc Anal Cytol. 2008;73(10):926–30. PubMed PMID: 18752282. Pubmed Central PMCID: 2773297.
67. Roederer M, Darzynkiewicz Z, Parks DR. Guidelines for the presentation of flow cytometric data. Methods Cell Biol. 2004;75:241–56.

Chapter 8
Lung Imaging in Animal Models

Emma Lefrançais, Beñat Mallavia and Mark R. Looney

Introduction

Animal models of lung injury and repair are designed to study inflammatory cell migration, cell signaling, and disruptions of the alveolar-capillary barrier. In vitro and ex vivo experiments, described in other chapters, have led to significant advances, but may involve the isolation and manipulation of cells that can affect their function. Cultured lung cells undergo phenotypic transformation, and terminal assays like histologic preparations, bronchoalveolar lavage, or cell sorting methods only provide a single snapshot in the evolution of the injury model. Even if the assays are useful in understanding what cells are present in the tissue and to quantify different parameters of lung injury, some important features like spatial and dynamic interactions can only be understood from live imaging. Lung imaging integrates the four dimensions of the tissue, one of time and three of space. Indeed, time is necessary to determine which physiologic processes are in progress or to estimate their rate. Lung imaging enables monitoring of the lung in its native setting and in real-time throughout the course of disease.

Lung Imaging Background

Lung Imaging Challenges and Peculiarities

Tissue microscopy has gained increased attention since the important advances in optical imaging technology. However, these methods were first applied to more

E. Lefrançais · B. Mallavia · M.R. Looney (✉)
Department of Medicine, University of California, San Francisco, San Francisco, CA, USA
e-mail: mark.looney@ucsf.edu

© Springer International Publishing AG 2017
L.M. Schnapp and C. Feghali-Bostwick (eds.), *Acute Lung Injury and Repair*,
Respiratory Medicine, DOI 10.1007/978-3-319-46527-2_8

accessible tissues, like the skin, cremaster muscle, or lymph nodes. The lung is probably one of the most difficult organs to observe under physiologic conditions as immobilization and exposure to the atmosphere interfere with its normal function. Indeed, imaging lung in vivo must overcome major obstacles. First, access to the organ requires opening of the chest wall, which leads to lung deflation without the intervention of positive pressure ventilation. Second, the motion due to both respiration and cardiac contractions further complicate the goal of a stable lung preparation. Next, the air-filled alveolar spaces pose an optical challenge, since air has a different refractive index than tissue. Lastly, the lung has a unique and delicate structure highly susceptible to mechanical and pro-inflammatory stress. These obstacles have been surmounted by different means including microscopic advancements, novel lung stabilization methods or the improvement of noninvasive imaging techniques. The lung is not only distinctive in its difficulty to image but also in its physiology. Indeed, the lung is the largest epithelial surface of the body in contact with the environment, the alveolar surface of the human lung being the size of a tennis court. Made for gas exchange, this area is also the site where potential pathogens meet one of the first lines of defense. Pulmonary circulation is peculiar as well, made of numerous interconnected capillary segments. These capillaries are particularly small, varying from 2 to 15 mm in diameter, which make the circulation of larger blood cells potentially difficult. Leukocyte sequestration and emigration mechanisms are consequently different from the systemic circulation. All these factors make lung imaging challenging and yet very promising to acquire unique knowledge.

History of Lung Imaging

The first microscopic observation of the lung was made in 1661 in Italy by Marcello Malpighi [1]. He was one of the first scientists to use the recently invented compound microscope, with an objective and an eyepiece lens. After failures using mammalian models, he used the frog and was the first person to observe and describe the lung capillaries and alveoli. His description completely changed perceptions of the structure of the lung that was thought to be similar to kidney or liver. He introduced for the first time the notion of vessels attached to an infinite number of air cavities. Two hundred fifty years later, Hall presented in 1925 a method for intravital microscopy of the lung in cats and rabbits [2]. To minimize respiratory movement he exteriorized a lobe out of the chest and fixed it with small clamps. However, exteriorization and fixation significantly alters the physiology of the lung and its circulation. To facilitate visual access to the lung in vivo, scientists then developed a series of increasingly refined thoracic window preparations. The first window was developed in the cat by Wearn et al. [3]. A window was excised in the thorax and the lung was transilluminated by creating a second window in the diaphragm through which the light beam of an arc lamp was passed. Curare was used to abolish respiratory movement and ventilation was maintained compressing the chest at short intervals. In 1939, Terry et al. [4, 5] constructed a thoracic window consisting of a metal cylinder mounted with a cover glass. Using cats, he inserted it in between two ribs and attached the microscope to the thoracic wall to follow respiration movement. To remove the air that entered the pleural cavity during surgery, he used an exhaust tube, allowing the lung to adhere to the cover glass. This window preparation permitted the observation of lung under closed thoracic conditions. Later, 1963, De Alva and Rainer [6] and Krahl [7] installed an intercostal window prosthesis in rabbit and dog that allowed observation of spontaneously breathing animals for several months. Mechanical ventilation was used during and after the surgery until spontaneous breathing was reestablished, removing air with a syringe. To manage the respiration movement, the microscope was focused at end-expiration or peak inspiration, which provided enough stabilization to acquire images. The thoracic window was improved by Wagner et al. [8] in **dogs** with a more elaborate suction system that was used to arrest cardiorespiratory movements allowing stable imaging of the live lung. The dogs were ventilated during the observation period.

Fluorescence-Based Imaging Techniques

Since the invention of the two lens microscope in the beginning of the seventieth century, advances in microscope technology have been considerable, improving image resolution, depth of imaging and sensitivity. Fluorescence microscopy is the technique that provides the highest spatial resolution among the available imaging techniques. We will describe briefly the microscopic techniques that enable live imaging and that can be used for lung imaging.

Microscopy Techniques Currently Used for Fluorescence Imaging

Imaging of a live tissue demands sufficient excitation energy to access to deep tissue layers but without creating photo damage. From conventional wide-field microscopy, to confocal and two-photon microscopy, the development of novel microscopy techniques has attempted to improve resolution (how much detail a user can observe, defined as the shortest distance between two points that a user can still see as separate images) and sensitivity (the ratio between signal to noise).

- *Wide-field microscopy*

In wide-field microscopy, the entire sample is excited with a specific band of wavelengths that matches the excitation of the fluorophore. The emitted signal is separated from the excitation light by specific filters. In this technique, fluorophore excitation is not restricted to the plane of focus, which causes image blur. It is therefore problematic to image structures deep below the surface or if stained structures are stacked on top of each other.

- *Confocal microscopy*

In confocal microscopy, the sample is excited by a laser which is focused to a single spot. Then, only the emitted signal from the focal plane is detected due to passage through a pinhole (Fig. 8.1a). Elimination of out of focus background leads to excellent spatial resolution and enables acquisition of images from within thick samples. Three-dimensional reconstructions can be produced when different illuminated planes are combined. However, during live imaging, a major drawback of confocal microscopy is that a large proportion of emitted light is discarded, blocked

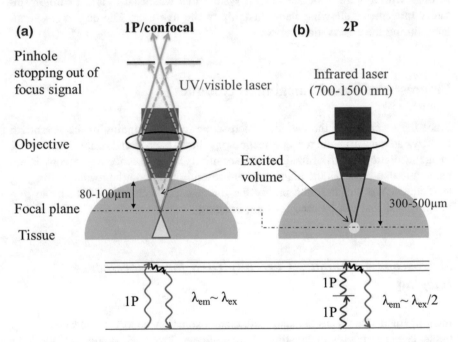

Fig. 8.1 Fluorescence microscopy imaging techniques used for intravital microscopy. **a** Confocal microscopy. (*Top*) In confocal microscopy, excitation and emission occur in a relative large volume around the focal plane (*yellow triangles*). The off-focus emissions are eliminated through a pinhole. (*Bottom*) In 1P microscopy, a fluorophore absorbs a single photon with a wavelength in the UV–visible range of the spectrum (*purple arrow*). After a vibrational relaxation (*black arrow*), a photon with a slightly shorter wavelength is emitted (*blue arrow*). Confocal microscopy enables imaging at a maximal depth to 80–100 μm. **b** Two-photon microscopy. (*Top*) Emission and excitation occur only at the focal plane in a restricted volume (*yellow spot*), and for this reason a pinhole is not required. (*Bottom*) In this process a fluorophore absorbs almost simultaneously two photons that have half of the energy (twice the wavelength) (*red arrow*) required for its excitation with a single photon. Two-photon excitations typically require IR light (from 700 to 1500 nm). Two-photon microscopy enables imaging at a maximal depth of 300–500 μm

by the pinhole. To establish sufficient sensitivity requires a strong excitation signal, which can cause photo damage and dye bleaching.

- **Two-photon microscopy**

The photo damage and bleaching that limit confocal microscopy can be overcome using two-photon (2P) microscopy. 2P excitation occurs when two lower energy photons (together having the equivalent energy of a single higher energy photon) are absorbed by a fluorophore. The probability of nearly simultaneous absorption of two photons is very low and will occur only at the focus of a high-energy pulsed laser (Fig. 8.2b). 2P is superior to confocal microscopy in the imaging of live tissues for two major reasons. First, only the point of focus is excited, inducing less photo damage and increasing the sensitivity. Second, the infrared excitation light used in 2P is less prone to scattering and penetrates deeper in living tissue, up to several hundred microns deep (compared with <80 μm with confocal). This makes it a very powerful technology for lung in vivo imaging.

Fig. 8.2 Examples of fluorescence intravital microscopy applications to study lung injury. Characteristics of acute lung injury are observed after intratracheal instillation with MRSA (Methicillin-resistant *Staphylococcus aureus* −5 × 10⁷ cfu). **a** Vascular permeability, observed by leakage into the alveolar space of i.v. Cascade Blue dextran. **b** Neutrophil elastase activity is monitored by the cleavage of a far red fluorescent substrate (NE680 FAST, Perkin Elmer), shown in pink in MRP8-Cre × mTmG lungs (GFP: neutrophils, tdTomato: ubiquitous). **c** Neutrophil recruitment is observed during the course of infection in MRP8-Cre × mTmG lungs at 3 and 5 h after infection. *White bars* indicate 30 μm

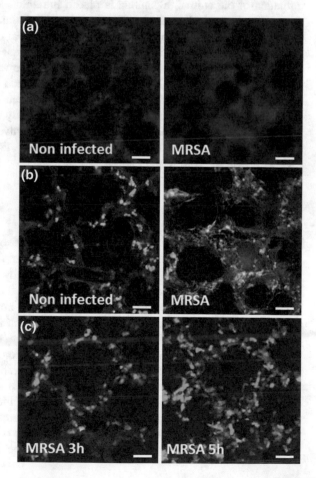

Lung Fluorescence Imaging Preparations

Technological advances in microscopy allow the acquisition of high-resolution images of the subpleural layers of the lung to analyze cellular and subcellular processes. Lung fluorescence imaging preparations can take three main forms: explanted tissues, live lungs slices placed under the flow of suitable medium, and intravital imaging where the lung is maintained in its natural microenvironment.

Live Lung Slices (LLS)

Description of LLS Preparation

The live lung slice method consists of partitioning the lung in thick slices, which are then carefully maintained to assure tissue viability. To do so, after the exsanguination of the animal, a cannula is placed intratracheally and lungs are inflated with 1.5–2 % liquid low melting agarose to maintain lung structure. The lungs are extracted and agarose is solidified in cold physiological medium. With the use of a micro-slicer or a vibratome, 150–300 μm thick serial slices are obtained. The vibration offers the possibility of cutting living tissue with a minimal injury. The slices are maintained in cell culture media at 37 °C and 5 % CO_2. Lung slices are normally used in the first 8 h although they have been used up to 2–3 days after sampling [9]. The lung slices have normal cell activity allowing the study of cell interactions and at the same time the structure of the alveoli is maintained to allow the 3D imaging of cell movements. For complete tissue preparation methods review, please see Thornton et al. [10].

Advantages and Disadvantages of LLS

LLS preparations have several advantages in comparison to fixed tissue imaging. First, fixed tissue samples are usually much thinner than live lung slices. The increased thickness of the live slices allows the study of three-dimensional cell movements that would be lost in thinner preparations or cellular monolayers. Second, and more importantly, unlike the static fixed images, LLS allow the study of time-dependent processes ranging from fast cell–cell interactions to the study of complex and slow pathogenic immune responses in the lung. Third, the LLS technique is a useful tool to study cellular interactions deep in the lung where intravital imaging or the isolated, perfused lung preparation cannot reach due to the excessive thickness. Because only a section of lung is studied with LLS preparations, it has important limitations such as the loss of blood and lymph circulation and the lack of neural input. These considerations are very important in studies requiring cell egress from other organs or other parts of the lung. Leukocyte activation induced by the isolation procedure may also be a concern.

Application of LLS in Lung Injury Studies

- *Cell death analysis*

In a work aimed to establish LLS as a suitable ex vivo technique to investigate the immunomodulatory effects and the characterization of cytokine production after LPS and other challenges, cell death was imaged by live/death fluorescence using confocal microscopy [9]. To distinguish living from dead cells, different dyes are used, such as Acridine Orange and Propidium Iodide. These markers allowed a better characterization of rat type II pneumocytes in an in situ patch clamp study [11]. TUNEL fluorescence analysis is also a very useful staining approach to study cell death. Jacobs et al. used this technique to study ROS-induced cell apoptosis [12].

- *Ca^{2+} measurement*

Pulmonary neuroephithelial bodies (NEB) are organized as clusters of pulmonary neuroendocrine cells during the development of the lung, and 4-Di-2-ASP fluorescent staining can be used to identify them in sliced lung preparations. Ca^{2+} signaling in the NEB microenvironment has been the focus of several studies. To facilitate imaging, Ca^{2+}-specific fluorescent dyes have been developed, from the commonly used Fluo-3 to its brighter analog Fluo-4. The use of these dyes allows real-time imaging of cellular Ca^{2+} flux using confocal microscopy [13, 14].

- *Tissue/cell identification*

The use of fluorescent antibodies in LLS preparations has improved protein and cellular identification due to the greater antigen accessibility compared with whole lung approaches. The use of Surfactant A and alveolar type II cell-specific antibodies allowed the identification of alveolar type II cells and the lamellar bodies contained within the cells [15].

- *Transgenic mouse studies*

The introduction of fluorescent markers opened the possibility to easily track and image target cell types or even cell subpopulations. Using a transgenic mouse where a yellow fluorescent protein expression is under the control of a promoter specific to antigen-presenting cells (CD11c-EYFP), Major Histocompatibility Complex (MHC) class II expression was studied. The lung slices were incubated with LPS and other pro-and anti-inflammatory molecules and the confocal fluorescence images showed that MHC-II expression was increased with pro-inflammatory challenges and repressed with dexamethasone [9].

Isolated, Perfused Lung Method (IPL)

Description of the IPL Method

In the isolated, perfused lung preparation, the left pulmonary artery is cannulated and perfused with autologous blood or a physiologic salt solution allowing passive drainage through the left ventricle. The lungs are ventilated with normal air or humidified gas containing different concentrations of oxygen and positive end-expiratory pressure is maintained. Using a perfusion pump, experimental agents can be added to the perfusate and introduced in the lung circulation. The lungs are suspended from a force displacement transducer to measure lung weight changes, while the whole system is maintained in a closed chamber with controlled humidity and temperature.

Advantages and Disadvantages of IPL

The main advantage of IPL technique over the live intravital approach is the unmatched stability of the sample. This important feature has permitted the use of directed microinjections of fluorescent dyes into endothelial or epithelial cell layers in the lungs [16]. Perfused whole lung preparations are a better approach to study lung physiology than LLS preparations. IPL preparations do not have the injured cut surfaces at the top and bottom of the preparation, which may induce undesirable effects when studying organ functionality. Vascular leakage is also better studied in isolated lungs than in LLS [17]. A clear disadvantage of isolated lung preparations is that it lacks the effects of the normal (or induced) physiological changes that occur systemically. This effect diminishes the possibility of leukocyte chemoattraction to the lungs from the bone marrow and circulation, which is an important limitation in inflammation-related studies. A possible leukocyte activation effect induced by the pump-assisted circulation used in the preparation of IPL is another disadvantage when compared with lung intravital microscopy [18].

Application of IPL to Lung Injury Models

• *Tissue/cell identification*

The labeling of mitochondria with fluorescent tags has allowed for the study of mitochondria transference in lung injury models. Islam et al. showed that mouse bone marrow-derived stromal cells, containing red fluorescent mitochondria, were located adjacent to epithelial cells minutes after their instillation into LPS-challenged isolated perfused lungs. In a further experiment, they showed by confocal microscopy that the fluorescent mitochondria were transferred to alveolar type II cells in a gap junction dependent process [19]. The use of other mitochondria markers (Mitotracker green, Ca^{2+} binding Rhod 2AM) allows their identification in endothelial cells [20].

• *Leukocyte trafficking*

Leukocytes are critical mediators of lung injury induced by endotoxemia, and the time that leukocytes spend in lung microvessels (venules and capillaries) depends on their activation state as well as the activation state of the endothelium. The use of fluorescence microscopy and R6G-rhodamine revealed that LPS-challenged microvessels retained leukocytes for a longer time than unchallenged lungs. The passage time is easily quantified in the surface vessels of isolated and perfused lungs without introducing any mechanical injury to the lungs [21].

- **ROS production**

Reactive oxygen species (ROS) production can be measured using fluorescence microscopy and the 2'–7'-dichlorodihydrofluoroscein acetate dye [20]. This technique was employed by Ichimura et al. to show that physical pressure-induced stress is able to promote ROS-triggered endothelial cell expression of P-selectin.

- **NO production**

Nitric oxide (NO) is a potent controller of the vascular tone in systemic and pulmonary vessels. Shear stress can promote the production of NO in endothelial cells. In 2000, in situ fluorescence procedures using IPL showed that shear stress was able to induce endothelial cell NO using a NO probe (diaminofluorescein diacetate), which was preceded by intracellular changes in Ca^{2+} detected using a fluorescent probe (Fluo-3) [22].

Lung Intravital Microscopy Methods (IVM)

Description of the Lung IVM Method

To observe the lung in a more physiological manner, it should be imaged in vivo. As discussed earlier, challenges faced with lung imaging compared to other organs are its intrinsic motion and the maintenance of breathing after opening the thorax. Different approaches have been developed to address these issues including (a) maintaining mechanical ventilation or reestablishment of spontaneous breathing, (b) the structure and composition of the window in contact with the lung, and (c) the management of cardiorespiratory motion.

- **Ventilation and closed thorax imaging**

Access to the lung requires opening of the thorax, which will cause lung collapse in the absence of positive pressure ventilation. Therefore, most of the preparations will use mechanical ventilation. Animals are anesthetized and tracheally intubated to be ventilated with room air or enriched oxygen. The animal is placed on a warming pad set to 37 °C to help maintain body temperature. To prevent dehydration, physiologic crystalloid solutions should be administered every hour or continuously. In some experiments, the thorax is closed after placing the window. To recover spontaneous breathing, the removal of the air introduced in the pleural cavity is required by vacuum or syringe suction. Mechanical ventilation is maintained until the lung is able to re-expand. Fingar et al. used a thoracic window implanted in rats to follow for 2 weeks the progression of pulmonary edema and alveolar flooding after lung injury by monitoring the leakage of vascular dyes [23]. Thoracic windows have been maintained in dog and rabbits for several months [6, 7]. Implanting a window has the advantage of not interfering with physiological respiration. However, because the motion is not controlled, it is not suited to high-resolution acquisition.

- **Thoracic windows specificities**

Once the thorax is open, it is important for high-resolution images to have stable windows with good optical properties and minimal interference with the normal structure and function of the lung. Most of the thoracic windows have used a metallic structure, first described by Terry et al. [4], to be introduced in between two adjacent ribs. The air from the pleural cavity is removed by suction or a syringe to bring the lung close to the observation window, which can be a cover glass [4, 24] or a transparent membrane made of Cronar [6] or Teflon [25]. To prevent the lung from dehydrating or cooling, the Teflon membrane used by Kuhnle et al. is covered by a warmed and bubbled Tyrode's solution. Metal and glass windows are efficient but their rigidity can induce trauma upon the delicate lung surface. Other approaches use less invasive methods, particularly in the mouse. Tabuchi et al. [26] used a polyvinylidene membrane sealed with glue over the ribs, and Kreisel et al. [27] attached the lung tissue to the bottom of a coverglass with tissue adhesive (VetBond). However, irritation may be produced from the moving lung touching the membrane potentially invoking an inflammatory response.

- **Control of lung motion**

One of the first approaches used on cats [3] and rats [23] was to use paralyzing agents to halt respiration. Another way to increase the time of stabilization is to temporarily suspend the respiration for 30 s [28] or in one of the two lungs by clamping the bronchus while ventilating the other lobe [29]. However, in these techniques where the respiration is blocked, the observed tissue will suffer from impaired oxygenation, which will undoubtedly affect the observed physiology. Without interrupting respiration, another technique has been to image the lung once every respiratory cycle, when the lung stops moving for a moment and comes back to the previous cycle position, at the end of the expiratory phase. This approach has been applied by Kuhnle et al. [25] and Tabuchi et al. [26]. This timing can be achieved by matching the ventilation rate and the acquisition. Indeed, imaging every 0.5 s with a ventilator rate of 120 breaths/min by Kreisel et al. [27] enables image acquisition once every breath cycle. More recently, in an effort to obtain more physiologic imaging, Fiole et al. did not use any stabilization procedure in the mouse lung during imaging, but instead corrected the images post hoc [30]. Every minute, a series of images was acquired and just one image was retained without any deformation. Lung structure was used as a frame of reference to select the correlated images by computer analysis.

Wagner et al. [8] addressed in an efficient way the obstacle of cardiorespiratory movement in live animal imaging using a thoracic window with built-in suction, providing enough stabilization for real-time microscopy. A similar technique, adapted from Wagner's thoracic window coupling suction to gently immobilize the lung on a glass coverslip has been recently adopted and miniaturized for mice by Looney et al. [24]. Different mouse windows were developed by groups in Germany [26], Japan [29] and USA [24, 27, 31]. The application of these lung intravital microscopy methods to mice has allowed access to the tools available with transgenic animals.

Advantages and Disadvantages of Intravital Microscopy

• *Advantages*

One advantage of fluorescence intravital microscopy is the high-resolution enabled by all fluorescent techniques. Compared to other techniques described for fluorescent imaging, lung intravital imaging makes it possible to observe lung injury under physiological conditions and with maintenance of the lung microenvironment. The preservation of blood and lymphatic circulation is one the main attractive features of IVM, which is important to study vascular permeability and leukocyte recruitment. It is consequently one of the most powerful approaches to study processes in lung injury animal models at a cellular and molecular scale.

• *Disadvantages*

One of the major limitations of intravital microscopy is the restricted ability to image deep in tissues. Imaging with two-photon excitation is confined mainly to 30–100 µm below the pleural surface, accessing only the most superficial layer of the lung. It may be a concern if the injury and inflammation in this superficial layer differ from the rest of the tissue. Moreover, the surgical preparation needed to access the lung could induce trauma that could have deleterious effects upon the microcirculation. Studies must be evaluated carefully considering the influences that may alter the normal physiology of the lung. Lastly, even though these IVM methods enable the acquisition of lung images up to several hours, it is currently unsuited for repeated observations in rodents.

Applications of IVM for Lung Injury Models

With these advanced fluorescence microscopy methods, it is possible to generate high-resolution images of several z-stack positions to generate 3D reconstitutions. The methods described also allow for imaging over several hours to generate time-lapsed data. It is then possible to analyze, localize, and quantify different parameters in four dimensions (3D plus time) such as cell velocity, colocalization, shape, volume, number, intensity, and color. Fluorescence is defined as the emission of light from a fluorescent probe after its excitation by an external light source of defined wavelength. The visualization of tissues, cells or proteins can be achieved by tagging molecules with specific fluorophores which can be selectively excited and specifically visualized. Here, we describe some useful applications for lung injury models.

- *Lung morphology and structural changes*

Visualizing the live lung enables the real-time observation of structural changes occurring during injury. For example, changes in lung vessel diameter by intravital microscopy was monitored during sepsis in rats [32] or after hypoxia in mice [26]. To visualize the lung structure several tools are available. Good resolution of the lung matrix can be obtained without using any extrinsic dyes due to the **second harmonic generation** effect. In a tissue, the specific molecular structure of collagen fibers generates an ultraviolet second harmonic light when excited with an infrared laser of a two-photon microscope. **Reporter mice ubiquitously expressing fluorescent proteins** also enable the imaging of stromal cells like the ubiquitously expressed actin-CFP reporter mice [29] or the mTmG reporter mice. A tdTomato fluorophore is expressed ubiquitously in the mTmG mice, and the localization of the fluorescent proteins to membrane structures outlines cell morphology and allows resolution of fine cellular processes (mT). This mouse can be crossed with a Cre-recombinase reporter mouse to target GFP expression in specific cell types (mG). Since the alveoli are surrounded by a dense meshwork of capillaries, **labeling of the blood circulation** by intravascular injection of tagged albumin, polysaccharides (dextran) or untargeted quantum-dots [33] will also produce an excellent outline of the alveolar structure.

- *Lung edema and vascular leakage*

Lung edema and vascular leakage is a characteristic feature of lung injury. Labeled albumin or labeled polysaccharides (dextran) injected intravenously can also be used to monitor vascular leakage in vivo. Indeed, under homeostatic conditions blood vessels limit the passage of dextran larger than 70 kDa, but during inflammatory conditions, dextran up to 2000 kDa can leak from the intravascular compartment [34]. Dextran efflux and vascular permeability can be quantified by measuring the changes in fluorescent intensity (Fig. 8.2a). The sensitivity of the fluorophore leakage can be modulated by using molecules of different sizes. Fingar et al. used a rat model of lung injury induced by oleic acid or compound 48/80 to directly measure in vivo the kinetics and magnitude of pulmonary vessel leakage and the development of edema. Leakage of intravascular FITC-albumin or rhodamine dye can be observed and quantified [23]. This same method was used to measure FITC dextran leakage after PMA or cigarette smoke-induced lung inflammation [31]. Looney et al. measured in mice the dynamic leakage of Texas Red dextran into the extravascular compartment during lung injury after intratracheal administration of LPS. Interestingly, in vivo imaging revealed a differential rate of vascular leakage across the imaged alveoli [24], an observation that could not have been made using measurement of global lung vascular permeability.

- *Leukocyte recruitment*

Another typical feature of lung injury is the rapid and massive recruitment of neutrophils into the lungs. Intravital microscopy is one of the most powerful techniques to study the anatomical location and dynamic influx of immune cells, and it is especially valuable for observing trafficking of cells from the circulation to peripheral tissues. Neutrophil recruitment into the lung is different from other vascular beds, and intravital microscopic approaches allow dissecting of these mechanisms in detail. Indeed, the size of a neutrophil (6–8 μm in diameter) can be bigger than the diameter of 50 % of the lung capillaries (2–15 μm). This may explain why neutrophils are sequestered in the lung. Sequestration of neutrophils has been observed in live rabbits by Kuebler et al. [35], and labeled leukocytes confirmed that lung capillaries are the predominant site of leukocyte sequestration. Neutrophil sequestration is accompanied by a morphological change into elongated shapes that have been observed in lung slices by actin labeling and confocal microscopy [36]. The same group made important discoveries about the requirement of selectins in sequestration and emigration of neutrophils in the lung [37]. Different tools are available to study neutrophils in vivo. Cells can be **isolated and fluorescently labeled with vital dyes** before infusion into recipient animals for fluorescence microscopy. Such a method was used by Presson et al. to observe the migration of Rhodamine-6G in vivo-labeled leukocytes into the rat lungs after PMA or cigarette smoke exposure [31]. The same group also demonstrated in a mouse IVM model the role of nitric oxide in neutrophil lung infiltration during sepsis using iNOS knockout mice [38]. Alternatively, the **injection of antibodies tagged** with a range of fluorescent dyes allows for labeling of neutrophils. However, caution must be taken when using this technique as antibodies can induce the activation or the depletion of the targeted cells. Anti-Gr-1, for example, can deplete neutrophils if high doses are used. In addition, the use of **transgenic mice expressing fluorescent proteins in a specific cell lineage** is a powerful method for specific labeling of leukocytes (Fig. 8.2c). A variety of strains have been created to track neutrophils. One example is the lysozyme-M (LysM)-green fluorescent protein (GFP) mouse that is characterized by bright green neutrophils and monocytes that are dim green. Using LysM-GFP mice, Kreisel et al. [27] observed by two-photon intravital imaging the mechanisms of neutrophil extravasation in bacterial pneumonia and ischemia-reperfusion after murine lung transplantation. A large pool of resident lung neutrophils was observed that rapidly increased in number after inflammatory challenge. Neutrophils clustered around monocytes, and the depletion of monocytes reduced this clustering phenomenon and reduced neutrophil extravasation. In the same mouse model of ischemia-reperfusion injury. They established that alveolar macrophages and their cell membrane associated protein DAP12 were important for the production of the chemokine CXCL2 and subsequent neutrophil extravasation [33]. However, LysM is expressed in the lung by both neutrophils and macrophages. To obtain fluorescent expression that is more restricted to neutrophils, the MRP8 promoter has been used [39]. Table 8.1 describes mouse strains commonly used to visualize cells in lung injury models.

Table 8.1 Fluorescent transgenic mice commonly used for lung injury models

Promoter/name	Reporter	Target cells
Lysozyme-M	GFP	Neutrophils, monocytes, macrophages
MRP8	GFP	Neutrophils
CX3CR1	GFP	Monocytes (low), macrophages (high), DC (int)
c-fms	YFP, GFP	Neutrophils, macrophages
CD11c	YFP	Dendritic cells, macrophages
PF4	tdTomato	Platelets
CD41	YFP	Platelets
Tie2	GFP	Blood vessels
Prox1	GFP	Lymphatic vessels
Actin	CFP	Ubiquitous
mTmG	tdTomato	Ubiquitous (membrane)
Lyn	Venus, GFP	Ubiquitous (membrane)

- *Dynamic cell-cell interactions*

The spatiotemporal observation of cell–cell interactions can stimulate new hypotheses about functional communications between cells and improve the understanding of lung inflammation. In a mouse model of lung injury after lung transplantation, Kreisel et al. [40] used CD11c-eYFP donor lungs transplanted into LysM-GFP recipient mice to observe direct interactions between donor dendritic cells and recipient neutrophils. These studies led to the discovery of a previously unknown link between neutrophils and DCs after lung transplantation that can explain the early events in lung inflammation. After *B. anthracis* pulmonary infection, the agent of anthrax, researchers also observed by IVM the interaction between DCs and alveolar macrophages using CX3CR1-GFP mice [30].

- *Protein staining and cellular functions*

Monitoring the expression of an important protein is also possible. Fingar et al. used the lung intravital method in rats to determine when and where in the pulmonary vasculature the adhesion molecule ICAM-1 was expressed after TNF-α-induced inflammation [28]. To be able to detect ICAM-1 binding sites under IVM, a two-step labeling procedure was used involving a monoclonal antibody against ICAM conjugated with fluorescent beads that generate enough fluorescence for detection. In addition, mice carrying reporters for cytokines such as IL-4 and interferon-γ have been made and can be used to image functional responses and cell fate decisions in real time.

- *Platelet biology*

The role of platelets during lung inflammation and injury has received increased attention in recent studies. The interaction of activated platelets with endothelium and neutrophils is important in influencing neutrophil sequestration and activation during the initial phases of lung injury. Lung intravital microscopy is an appropriate method to investigate the dynamics and mechanisms of these heterotypic interactions. Methods to label platelets include using transgenic animals (CD41-YFP, PF4-tdTomato) and fluorescent monoclonal antibodies (CD49b, CD42b). Intravital microscopy studies in rabbit [41] and mouse [26] showed the retention of labeled platelets in the lung microcirculation after their activation. Using mice obtained by crossing PF4-tdTomato with LysM-GFP mice, our group was able to visualize by 2-photon IVM the real-time interactions between neutrophils and platelets in LPS-induced lung injury. Neutrophil-platelet aggregates in the lung circulation were observed under homeostatic conditions and their number greatly increased after LPS challenge, including in the alveolar spaces, and could be reduced after aspirin treatment, concomitantly with lung injury reduction [42].

- *Protease activity (fluorescent substrates)*

Inflammatory proteases, such as neutrophil elastase, have been implicated in the pathophysiology of acute lung injury. Specific protease substrates can be used as activatable reporter probes to localize and quantify protease activity in real time. Cleavage of the probe leads to the liberation of the fluorophore. Elastase [43], MMP [44] and Cathepsin [45]-sensitive probes can be used for a better understanding of protease activity during lung inflammation (Fig. 8.2b).

- *Cell death, injury, and extracellular DNA*

Lung injury is accompanied by endothelial and epithelial cell death. It can be monitored by the use of cell membrane-impermeable cyanine nucleic acid dyes, which only stain dead cells. Neutrophil activation has been involved in cell injury, but the role of cytotoxic proteases in this cell toxicity is still not clear. Recently, neutrophils have been shown to release in the extracellular space their DNA, covered with neutrophil proteases. These neutrophil extracellular traps (NETs) are believed to serve as an antibacterial defense mechanism. However, data suggest that NETs can, in the delicate lung microcirculation, contribute to lung endothelial injury [46]. NETs, made of characteristic DNA strands, can be stained in vivo with cell impermeable nucleotide dyes [47]. Intravital microscopy could reveal the presence and localization of NETs during lung injury and inform their interaction in situ with leukocytes, platelets, and endothelial/epithelial cells.

Noninvasive Imaging Techniques

Bioluminescence Imaging (BLI)

Principles of Luminescence Imaging

Bioluminescence imaging (BLI) is based on the sensitive detection of visible light produced during a biochemical reaction. The oxidation of the substrate luciferin, in presence of ATP, is catalyzed by the expression of the enzyme luciferase, leading to the emission of light at 560 nm. The luciferase enzyme is naturally found in the firefly, but can be artificially incorporated into cells and animal models under the control of specific promoters. Light from the cells that express the luciferase reporter gene can then be detected when the appropriate substrate is added. The IVIS imaging system consists of a CCD camera mounted on top of a light impermeable chamber where the animal is placed. A heating stage and anesthetics keep the animal warm and sedated. This imaging modality has proven to be a very powerful methodology to detect luciferase reporter activity in intact animal models.

Advantages and Disadvantages of BLI

BLI is low-cost, noninvasive, and facilitates real-time analysis of lung injury processes at the molecular level in living organisms. Since it is noninvasive, each animal can be imaged at multiple time points. BLI allows acquisition of the whole mouse lung, since it is possible to image as deep as several centimeters within tissue. However, compared to fluorescent methods, the resolution is lower and inflammation can only be localized to the organ level. The sensitivity of the NF-κB luciferase reporter mouse has been questioned in the study of lung inflammation by Hadina et al. [48]. It was demonstrated that low-dose LPS was not able to induce any detectable bioluminescence and was therefore less sensitive than measuring neutrophils or cytokines in lung lavage. A significant and quantifiable signal was detectable in the lungs after an intranasal LPS dose of 1.2 mg/kg. Also, quantitative analysis must be approached with caution since light emission depends on the activity of the promoter gene of interest and on the presence of ATP, oxygen and the substrate. The intensity of light is also dependent on the depth of the labeled cells, since light has to travel through the tissue.

Application of BLI in Lung Injury Models

Bioluminescence provides a noninvasive method to monitor gene expression in vivo. Depending on the targeted gene, BLI can serve different purposes.

- *NF-κB/luciferase reporter mice*

One of the most extensively used luminescent reporter animals is a transgenic mouse expressing the firefly luciferase under the control of a NF-κB-dependent promoter. These mice enable a quantitative method for evaluating the localization, the timing, and the level of NF-κB activation in vivo during inflammatory models. These mice have been used in lung injury models induced by LPS, *Pseudomonas aeruginosa* [49], TNF-alpha or IL-1beta [50]. This strain is also useful to test if specific interventions or anti-inflammatory therapies [51, 52] can affect the inflammation that is dependent on NF-κB activity. In the lung, Sadikot et al. showed that the host response to *P. aeruginosa* can be altered in the lung epithelium in vivo using adenoviral vectors to activate or inhibit NF-κB [53].

- **ROS generation and MPO activity by luminol or lucigerin substrate**

Another bioluminescent chemical reaction used is the oxidation of luminol or lucigenin substrate catalyzed by the presence of reactive oxygen species (ROS). ROS play an important role in lung injury, and delineating in real time their generation and contribution can be done using luminescent substrates without the use of transgenic mice. In a lung inflammation model induced by intratracheal zymosan, Han et al. [54] demonstrated increased ROS levels in WT but not in $p47^{phox-/-}$ mice, indicating that NADPH oxidase is the major source of ROS generation. Luminol and lucigenin bioluminescent reactions depend on different ROS species. Neutrophil MPO is involved in luminol conversion and can be used to image acute inflammation and neutrophil enriched areas. Lucigenin biolumines-cence can be used to detect NADPH activity from macrophages [55].

- **Inflammatory cell migration and bacterial load**

The introduction of a luciferase reporter gene into T cells [56], macrophages [57], or other immune cells can be used to follow the trafficking of these cells in lung inflammation and injury models. It can be useful in infectious models of lung injury to monitor the bacterial load in the lung or the circulation. This can be achieved by tracking bioluminescent strains of bacteria (*P. aeruginosa* [49], *S. pneumoniae* [58], *S. aureus* [59], *H. influenza* [60]).

Magnetic Resonance Imaging (MRI)

Principles of MRI

Magnetic Resonance Imaging (MRI) is a noninvasive imaging technique that uses a strong magnetic field and radio waves to excite protons contained in different tissues. When the excited protons realign, they emit a radio frequency absorbed by a receiving coil that allows generation of an image of the tissue.

Advantages and Disadvantages of MRI

One of the biggest advantages of this imaging technique is the absence of ionizing radiation, allowing repeated measurements without risking injury to the lungs. In general, however, lung imaging presents two major problems to the use of magnetic resonance image techniques. Motion induced by respiration is the first problem, which can be improved by synchronized ventilation. The second problem is the reduced discriminating capacity of the air-tissue interface due to high water and air content in lungs, leading to a reduced signal. To improve the resolution, the clas-sical proton MRI has been improved by the addition of ultra-short eco time, which has not only increased the resolution but also reduced the imaging time [61, 62].

The use of hyperpolarized ^{129}Xe and most recently, ^{3}He gas has also drastically increased MRI capability to study structural and functional characteristics of the lungs [63, 64]. The use of contrast agents has propelled MRI imaging to a new level of functionality. Ogasawara et al. showed in a radiation-induced lung injury model in dogs that the addition of a contrast agent (gadolinium-DTPA) allowed the discernment of different radiation pneumonitis phases [65].

Applications of MRI in Lung Injury Models

Experimental acute lung injury revealed that inflammation areas localized by MRI correlated with histological and pathological analyses in an IL1β + TNFα instillation model [66]. High-resolution MRI was used by Bosmann et al. to show the effect of extracellular histones in three different ALI models. Histone presence correlated with lung injury observed in the MR images [67]. MRI was more sensitive than high-resolution computed tomography (HR-CT) for the detection of early pathologic changes induced by hyperoxia [68].

Radiation-Based Imaging Techniques: Micro-CT

Principles of Micro-CT

Micro-Computerized Tomography (CT) imaging utilizes X-rays to form virtual slices that are transformed in 2D or 3D images by the software. The signal that is measured in Hounsfield units (HU) depends on the decay of the x-rays when they cross different tissues. The air has a value of -1000 and water a value of 0.

Advantages and Disadvantages of Micro-CT

This noninvasive technique has the inconvenience of the ionizing radiation that may prevent its repeated use in a short period of time. Although Chandra et al. suggested that the radiation used in CT might have an effect on bone loss [69], other studies suggest that the low dose used does not have any cardiopulmonary effect [70]. The main advantage compared to classical x-rays is the serial acquisition of the images allowing a 3D reconstruction that is more informative than a 2D image. CT imaging is also cheaper and faster than MRI. Computer tomography can be used in studies involving metallic implants, which is not possible with MRI. Respiration-gated micro-CT has solved some of the motion problems relevant to live lung imaging. The use of a faster flat-panel volumetric CT has reduced the acquisition time to a few seconds [71].

Applications of Micro-CT in Lung Injury Models

In a dog model of LPS-induced acute lung injury, the use of computed tomography showed vascular leak and edema formation. In this study, the injection of sphingosine 1-phosphate reduced the vascular leak [72]. In an oleic acid-induced lung injury model, pulmonary parenchymal infiltrates were visible using micro-CT [73]. By measuring lung volumes radiographically at end-inspiration and end-expiration, pulmonary compliance can be calculated using computed tomography. Bleomycin challenge reduced lung compliance (measured by CT) in a mouse model [74]. In a similar model of ALI induced by oleic acid, Perchiazzi et al. demonstrated reduced lung compliance in the injured mice [75]. Finally, Fernandez-Bustillo observed using a LPS-induced ALI model that increased IL-1β levels in BAL correlated with an increase in apex-base CT-derived compliance differences [76].

Radiation-Based Imaging Techniques: PET/SPECT

Principles of PET/SPECT

Gamma ray emission imaging techniques are based on the use of small radiolabeled molecules (tracers) that are injected in the body while a gamma camera records the signal they emit. Positron emission tomography (PET) measures 2 gamma photons emitted in 180° angle separation after the positron emitted by the tracer collides against an electron in the tissue. On the other hand, single photon emission computed tomography (SPECT) measures single gamma rays emitted by the tracer.

Advantages and Disadvantages of PET/SPECT

The need of a collimator in SPECT imaging reduces the sensitivity and increases the number of artifacts acquired comparing with PET imaging. But the shorter half-life of the isotopes used in PET (typically Fluorine-18) when compared with the isotopes used in SPECT (Thalium-201 or Technetium-99 m), reduces their availability and increases their price. Both techniques use ionizing radiation, which can be deleterious in sequential acquisitions. PET and SECT imaging can be integrated with high-resolution CT imaging to allow the correlation of functional and metabolic abnormalities with morphological features in the lung [77].

Applications of PET/SPECT in Lung Injury Models

Mintun studied vascular permeability induced by oleic acid in a dog lung injury model and showed that gallium-68 labeled transferrin leaked more into the extravascular space in challenged than in unchallenged lungs [78]. More recently the tracer used in lung injury models has changed to [^{18}F]-flouro-2-deoxy-D-glucose (18F-FDG). This glucose-derived tracer labeled with Fluorine-18, is the principal tracer used in PET scans to analyze lung injury and it is internalized by the glucose transporter-1. FDG used as leukocyte marker, facilitates the study of neutrophil and macrophage recruitment in the lungs. PET scan studies show that the infiltration peak induced by hydrochloric acid is 24–48 h after instillation [79]. FDG can also be used to determine the activation state of neutrophils measured by their uptake of this tracer. PET/CT with 18F-FDG allows the assessment of both lung aeration and neutrophil inflammation as well as an estimation of the regional fraction of blood. Pouzot et al. used this method to validate the use of regional fraction of blood to assess pulmonary blood flow, using PET in both control animals and animals with ALI [80]. SPECT imaging has been used to study endothelial cell death in a hyperoxia model of ALI [81], and it is useful to analyze the alterations of regional blood flow in saline lavaged lungs [82] or lungs treated with oleic acid [83].

Conclusions and Future Directions

Imaging of live tissues, such as the lung, is being increasingly applied to the study of disease processes, and the importance of combining and confirming data with an imaging technique is becoming more common. More importantly, live imaging also provides the opportunity for relevant observations and discoveries that could not have been done by other ex vivo or static methods. In this chapter, we have described different techniques for imaging the lung, illustrating advantages and limitations of the various methods. The recent adaptation of the intravital micro-scopy technique to the mouse lung has been a step forward for the field and holds much promise. Combined with two-photon fluorescence microscopy, it is probably the best technique to enable imaging of the lung in real time and its natural envi-ronment. As lung intravital microscopy is still limited by imaging depth below the pleural surface, an alternative can be the preparation of lung slices for live imaging. The high-resolution of both techniques supports cellular and molecular-scaled analysis like cell interactions and dynamics. Depending on the level of resolution required for the application, other noninvasive methods can be used for morpho-logical studies (MRI, Micro-CT) or functional studies (Bioluminescence, PET/SPECT). Table 8.2 summarizes the parameters important in choosing an imaging technique for biological application.

We described for each method several applications in the scope of lung injury research. We expect that the increasing availability of transgenic mice and molecular reagent to label cells and their subtypes will bring new applications for animal models. Improvement in lung imaging could also be produced through technical advances in microscopy. Confocal and two-photon microscopy require invasive preparations to access the organ, which is particularly challenging for the

Table 8.2 Lung imaging methods. Overview of the methods used in live lung imaging

		Resolution	Application	Imaging depth	Physiological environment	Invasivity
Fluorescence	Lung slices (LLS)	<1 μm	Molecular scale imaging (cells, protein,…)	100 μm (deep layers of the lung accessible)	Ex vivo	Tissue isolated and sectioned
	Perfused Lung (IPL)	<1 μm	Molecular scale imaging (cells, protein,…)	100 μm	Ex vivo-*whole organ*	Isolated tissue
	Intravital (IVM)	<1 μm	Molecular scale imaging (cells, protein,…)	100 μm	In vivo	Surgery required
Bioluminescence		1 mm	Functional imaging (reporter genes)	Whole body	In vivo	Noninvasive
MRI		100 μm	Lung structure	Whole body	In vivo	Noninvasive
Micro-CT		1 μm	Lung structure	Whole body	In vivo	Noninvasive
PET/SPECT		1 mm	Functional imaging (cell activity)	Whole body	In vivo	Noninvasive

lung. Miniaturization of confocal and two-photon microscopes has been developed and is being optimized [84]. The use of confocal endoscopy has been described in the lung [85, 86] and a miniaturized endoscope with an outer diameter of 0.75 mm can be inserted into the animal through a small keyhole incision or through the main bronchi of the mouse [87]. Such an application could address the idealized lung imaging technique—one that produces high-resolution and non- or minimally-invasive in vivo imaging.

References

1. Young J. Malpighi's "De Pulmonibus". Proceedings of the Royal Society of Medicine. 1929;23(1):1–11 (Epub 1929/11/01).
2. Hall HL. A study of the pulmonary circulation by the trans-illumination method. Am J Physiol. 1925;72:446–57.
3. Wearn JT, Ernestene AC, Bromer AW, Barr JW, German WJ, Zschiesche LJ. The normal behavior of the pulmonary blood vessels with observations on the intermittence of the flow of blood in arterioles and capillaries. Am J Physiol. 1934;109:236–56.
4. Terry RJ. A thoracic window for observation of the lung in a living animal. Science. 1939;90 (2324):43–4 (Epub 1939/07/14).
5. Terry RJ. The presence of water on the respiratory surfaces of the lung. Am J Anat. 1964;115:559–68 (Epub 1964/11/01).
6. De Alva WE, Rainer WG. A method of high speed in vivo pulmonary microcinematography under physiologic conditions. Angiology. 1963;14:160–4 (Epub 1963/04/01).
7. Krahl VE. A method of studying the living lung in the closed thorax, and some preliminary observations. Angiology. 1963;14:149–59 (Epub 1963/04/01).
8. Wagner WW Jr. Pulmonary microcirculatory observations in vivo under physiological conditions. J Appl Physiol. 1969;26(3):375–7 (Epub 1969/03/01).
9. Henjakovic M, Sewald K, Switalla S, Kaiser D, Muller M, Veres TZ, et al. Ex vivo testing of immune responses in precision-cut lung slices. Toxicol Appl Pharmacol. 2008;231(1):68–76 (Epub 2008/05/28).
10. Thornton EE, Krummel MF, Looney MR. Live imaging of the lung. Curr Protoc Cytom. 2012;Chap. 12:Unit12 28.
11. Shlyonsky V, Goolaerts A, Mies F, Naeije R. Electrophysiological characterization of rat type II pneumocytes in situ. Am J Respir Cell Mol Biol. 2008;39(1):36–44 (Epub 2008/02/16).
12. Jacobs ER, Bodiga S, Ali I, Falck AM, Falck JR, Medhora M, et al. Tissue protection and endothelial cell signaling by 20-HETE analogs in intact ex vivo lung slices. Exp Cell Res. 2012;318(16):2143–52 Epub 2012/06/13.
13. Lembrechts R, Brouns I, Schnorbusch K, Pintelon I, Kemp PJ, Timmermans JP, et al. Functional expression of the multimodal extracellular calcium-sensing receptor in pulmonary neuroendocrine cells. J Cell Sci. 2013;126(Pt 19):4490–501 (Epub 2013/07/28).
14. Schnorbusch K, Lembrechts R, Pintelon I, Timmermans JP, Brouns I, Adriaensen D. GABAergic signaling in the pulmonary neuroepithelial body microenvironment: functional imaging in GAD67-GFP mice. Histochem Cell Biol. 2013;140(5):549–66 (Epub 2013/04/10).
15. Helms MN, Jain L, Self JL, Eaton DC. Redox regulation of epithelial sodium channels examined in alveolar type 1 and 2 cells patch-clamped in lung slice tissue. J Biol Chem. 2008;283(33):22875–83 (Epub 2008/06/11).
16. Looney MR, Bhattacharya J. Live imaging of the lung. Annu Rev Physiol. 2014;76:431–45 (Epub 2013/11/20).

17. Chouteau JM, Obiako B, Gorodnya OM, Pastukh VM, Ruchko MV, Wright AJ, et al. Mitochondrial DNA integrity may be a determinant of endothelial barrier properties in oxidant-challenged rat lungs. Am J Physiol Lung Cell Mol Physiol. 2011;301(6):L892–8 (Epub 2011/09/06).

18. Baufreton C, Kirsch M, Loisance DY. Measures to control blood activation during assisted circulation. Ann Thorac Surg. 1998;66:1837–44.

19. Islam MN, Das SR, Emin MT, Wei M, Sun L, Westphalen K, et al. Mitochondrial transfer from bone-marrow-derived stromal cells to pulmonary alveoli protects against acute lung injury. Nat Med. 2012;18(5):759–65 (Epub 2012/04/17).

20. Ichimura H, Parthasarathi K, Quadri S, Issekutz AC, Bhattacharya J. Mechano-oxidative coupling by mitochondria induces proinflammatory responses in lung venular capillaries. J Clin Invest. 2003;111(5):691–9.

21. Kandasamy K, Sahu G, Parthasarathi K. Real-time imaging reveals endothelium-mediated leukocyte retention in LPS-treated lung microvessels. Microvasc Res. 2012;83(3):323–31 Epub 2012/02/22.

22. Al-Mehdi AB, Song C, Tozawa K, Fisher AB. Ca^{2+}- and PI3 kinase-dependent nitric oxide generation in lung endothelial cells in situ with ischemia. J Biol Chem. 2000;275(51):39807–10.

23. Fingar VH, Taber SW, Wieman TJ. A new model for the study of pulmonary microcirculation: determination of pulmonary edema in rats. J Surg Res. 1994;57(3):385–93 Epub 1994/09/01.

24. Looney MR, Thornton EE, Sen D, Lamm WJ, Glenny RW, Krummel MF. Stabilized imaging of immune surveillance in the mouse lung. Nat Methods. 2011;8(1):91–6 Epub 2010/12/15.

25. Kuhnle GE, Leipfinger FH, Goetz AE. Measurement of microhemodynamics in the ventilated rabbit lung by intravital fluorescence microscopy. J Appl Physiol (1985). 1993;74(3):1462–71 (Epub 1993/03/01).

26. Tabuchi A, Mertens M, Kuppe H, Pries AR, Kuebler WM. Intravital microscopy of the murine pulmonary microcirculation. J Appl Physiol (1985). 2008;104(2):338–46 (Epub 2007/11/17).

27. Kreisel D, Nava RG, Li W, Zinselmeyer BH, Wang B, Lai J, et al. In vivo two-photon imaging reveals monocyte-dependent neutrophil extravasation during pulmonary inflammation. Proc Natl Acad Sci USA. 2010;107(42):18073–8 Epub 2010/10/07.

28. Fingar VH, Taber SW, Buschemeyer WC, ten Tije A, Cerrito PB, Tseng M, et al. Constitutive and stimulated expression of ICAM-1 protein on pulmonary endothelial cells in vivo. Microvasc Res. 1997;54(2):135–44 Epub 1997/11/05.

29. Hasegawa A, Hayashi K, Kishimoto H, Yang M, Tofukuji S, Suzuki K, et al. Color-coded real-time cellular imaging of lung T-lymphocyte accumulation and focus formation in a mouse asthma model. J Allergy Clin Immunol. 2010;125(2):461–8 e6 (Epub 2009/12/25).

30. Fiole D, Deman P, Trescos Y, Mayol JF, Mathieu J, Vial JC, et al. Two-photon intravital imaging of lungs during anthrax infection reveals long-lasting macrophage-dendritic cell contacts. Infect Immun. 2014;82(2):864–72 Epub 2014/01/31.

31. Presson RG Jr, Brown MB, Fisher AJ, Sandoval RM, Dunn KW, Lorenz KS, et al. Two-photon imaging within the murine thorax without respiratory and cardiac motion artifact. Am J Pathol. 2011;179(1):75–82 Epub 2011/06/28.

32. McCormack DG, Mehta S, Tyml K, Scott JA, Potter R, Rohan M. Pulmonary microvascular changes during sepsis: evaluation using intravital videomicroscopy. Microvasc Res. 2000;60 (2):131–40 Epub 2000/08/31.

33. Spahn JH, Li W, Bribriesco AC, Liu J, Shen H, Ibricevic A, et al. DAP12 expression in lung macrophages mediates ischemia/reperfusion injury by promoting neutrophil extravasation. J Immunol. 2015;194(8):4039–48 Epub 2015/03/13.

34. Egawa G, Nakamizo S, Natsuaki Y, Doi H, Miyachi Y, Kabashima K. Intravital analysis of vascular permeability in mice using two-photon microscopy. Sci Rep. 2013;3:1932 (Epub 2013/06/05).

35. Kuebler WM, Kuhnle GE, Groh J, Goetz AE. Leukocyte kinetics in pulmonary microcir-culation: intravital fluorescence microscopic study. J Appl Physiol (1985). 1994;76(1):65–71 (Epub 1994/01/01).

36. Motosugi H, Graham L, Noblitt TW, Doyle NA, Quinlan WM, Li Y, et al. Changes in neutrophil actin and shape during sequestration induced by complement fragments in rabbits. Am J Pathol. 1996;149(3):963–73 Epub 1996/09/01.

37. Doyle NA, Bhagwan SD, Meek BB, Kutkoski GJ, Steeber DA, Tedder TF, et al. Neutrophil margination, sequestration, and emigration in the lungs of L-selectin-deficient mice. J Clin Investig. 1997;99(3):526–33 Epub 1997/02/01.

38. Razavi HM, le Wang F, Weicker S, Rohan M, Law C, McCormack DG, et al. Pulmonary neutrophil infiltration in murine sepsis: role of inducible nitric oxide synthase. Am J Respir Crit Care Med. 2004;170(3):227–33 Epub 2004/04/03.

39. Passegue E, Wagner EF, Weissman IL. JunB deficiency leads to a myeloproliferative disorder arising from hematopoietic stem cells. Cell. 2004;119(3):431–43 Epub 2004/10/28.

40. Kreisel D, Sugimoto S, Zhu J, Nava R, Li W, Okazaki M, et al. Emergency granulopoiesis promotes neutrophil-dendritic cell encounters that prevent mouse lung allograft acceptance. Blood. 2011;118(23):6172–82 Epub 2011/10/06.

41. Eichhorn ME, Ney L, Massberg S, Goetz AE. Platelet kinetics in the pulmonary microcirculation in vivo assessed by intravital microscopy. J Vasc Res. 2002;39(4):330–9 Epub 2002/08/21.

42. Ortiz-Munoz G, Mallavia B, Bins A, Headley M, Krummel MF, Looney MR. Aspirin-triggered 15-epi-lipoxin A4 regulates neutrophil-platelet aggregation and attenuates acute lung injury in mice. Blood. 2014;124(17):2625–34 (Epub 2014/08/22).

43. Kossodo S, Zhang J, Groves K, Cuneo GJ, Handy E, Morin J, et al. Noninvasive in vivo quantification of neutrophil elastase activity in acute experimental mouse lung injury. Int J Mol Imaging. 2011;2011:581406 Epub 2011/09/24.

44. Bremer C, Tung CH, Weissleder R. In vivo molecular target assessment of matrix metalloproteinase inhibition. Nat Med. 2001;7(6):743–8 Epub 2001/06/01.

45. Haller J, Hyde D, Deliolanis N, de Kleine R, Niedre M, Ntziachristos V. Visualization of pulmonary inflammation using noninvasive fluorescence molecular imaging. J Appl Physiol (1985). 2008;104(3):795–802 (Epub 2008/01/19).

46. Caudrillier A, Kessenbrock K, Gilliss BM, Nguyen JX, Marques MB, Monestier M, et al. Platelets induce neutrophil extracellular traps in transfusion-related acute lung injury. J Clin Invest. 2012;122(7):2661–71.

47. Kolaczkowska E, Jenne CN, Surewaard BG, Thanabalasuriar A, Lee WY, Sanz MJ, et al. Molecular mechanisms of NET formation and degradation revealed by intravital imaging in the liver vasculature. Nat Commun. 2015;6:6673 Epub 2015/03/27.

48. Hadina S, Wohlford-Lenane CL, Thorne PS. Comparison of in vivo bioluminescence imaging and lavage biomarkers to assess pulmonary inflammation. Toxicology. 2012;291(1–3):133–8 Epub 2011/12/03.

49. Sadikot RT, Zeng H, Yull FE, Li B, Cheng DS, Kernodle DS, et al. p47phox deficiency impairs NF-kappa B activation and host defense in Pseudomonas pneumonia. J Immunol. 2004;172(3):1801–8 Epub 2004/01/22.

50. Carlsen H, Moskaug JO, Fromm SH, Blomhoff R. In vivo imaging of NF-kappa B activity. J Immunol. 2002;168(3):1441–6 (Epub 2002/01/22).

51. Sadikot RT, Jansen ED, Blackwell TR, Zoia O, Yull F, Christman JW, et al. High-dose dexamethasone accentuates nuclear factor-kappa b activation in endotoxin-treated mice. Am J Respir Crit Care Med. 2001;164(5):873–8 Epub 2001/09/11.

52. Kim KH, Kwun MJ, Choi JY, Ahn KS, Oh SR, Lee YG, et al. Therapeutic effect of the tuber of alisma orientale on lipopolysaccharide-induced acute lung injury. Evid-Based Complement Altern Med: eCAM. 2013;2013:863892 (Epub 2013/08/29).

53. Sadikot RT, Zeng H, Joo M, Everhart MB, Sherrill TP, Li B, et al. Targeted immunomod-ulation of the NF-kappaB pathway in airway epithelium impacts host defense against Pseudomonas aeruginosa. J Immunol. 2006;176(8):4923–30 (Epub 2006/04/06).

54. Han W, Li H, Segal BH, Blackwell TS. Bioluminescence imaging of NADPH oxidase activity in different animal models. J Visualized Exp: JoVE. 2012(68) (Epub 2012/11/03).

55. Tseng JC, Kung AL. In vivo imaging of inflammatory phagocytes. Chem Biol. 2012;19 (9):1199–209 Epub 2012/09/25.

56. Dugger KJ, Chrisman T, Jones B, Chastain P, Watson K, Estell K, et al. Moderate aerobic exercise alters migration patterns of antigen specific T helper cells within an asthmatic lung. Brain Behav Immun. 2013;34:67–78 Epub 2013/08/10.

57. Lee HW, Jeon YH, Hwang MH, Kim JE, Park TI, Ha JH, et al. Dual reporter gene imaging for tracking macrophage migration using the human sodium iodide symporter and an enhanced firefly luciferase in a murine inflammation model. Mol Imaging Biol: MIB: Official Publication the Acad Mol Imaging. 2013;15(6):703–12 Epub 2013/05/17.

58. Francis KP, Yu J, Bellinger-Kawahara C, Joh D, Hawkinson MJ, Xiao G, et al. Visualizing pneumococcal infections in the lungs of live mice using bioluminescent Streptococcus pneumoniae transformed with a novel gram-positive lux transposon. Infect Immun. 2001;69 (5):3350–8 Epub 2001/04/09.

59. Francis KP, Joh D, Bellinger-Kawahara C, Hawkinson MJ, Purchio TF, Contag PR. Monitoring bioluminescent Staphylococcus aureus infections in living mice using a novel luxABCDE construct. Infect Immun. 2000;68(6):3594–600 Epub 2000/05/19.

60. Jurcisek JA, Bookwalter JE, Baker BD, Fernandez S, Novotny LA, Munson RS Jr, et al. The PilA protein of non-typeable Haemophilus influenzae plays a role in biofilm formation, adherence to epithelial cells and colonization of the mammalian upper respiratory tract. Mol Microbiol. 2007;65(5):1288–99 (Epub 2007/07/25).

61. Egger C, Cannet C, Gerard C, Jarman E, Jarai G, Feige A, et al. Administration of bleomycin via the oropharyngeal aspiration route leads to sustained lung fibrosis in mice and rats as quantified by UTE-MRI and histology. PLoS One. 2013;8(5):e63432 (Epub 2013/05/15).

62. Wurnig MT, Y; Weiger, M; Jungraithmayr, W; Boss, A. Assessing lung transplantation ischemia-reperfusion injury by microcomputed tomography and ultrashort echo-time magnetic resonance imaging in a mouse model. Invest Radiol. 2013;49(1):23–8.

63. Rudolph A, Markstaller K, Gast KK, David M, Schreiber WG, Eberle B. Visualization of alveolar recruitment in a porcine model of unilateral lung lavage using ^{3}He-MRI. Acta Anaesthesiol Scand. 2009;53(10):1310–6 (Epub 2009/08/18).

64. Thomas AC, Nouls JC, Driehuys B, Voltz JW, Fubara B, Foley J, et al. Ventilation defects observed with hyperpolarized ^{3}He magnetic resonance imaging in a mouse model of acute lung injury. Am J Respir Cell Mol Biol. 2011;44(5):648–54 Epub 2010/07/03.

65. Ogasawara NS, K; Karino, Y; Matsunaga, N. Perfusion characteristics of radiation-injured lung on Gd-DTPA-enhanced dynamic magnetic resonance imaging. Invest Radiol. 2002;37 (8):448–57.

66. Serkova NJ, Van Rheen Z, Tobias M, Pitzer JE, Wilkinson JE, Stringer KA. Utility of magnetic resonance imaging and nuclear magnetic resonance-based metabolomics for quantification of inflammatory lung injury. Am J Physiol Lung Cell Mol Physiol. 2008;295 (1):L152–61 Epub 2008/04/29.

67. Bosmann M, Grailer JJ, Ruemmler R, Russkamp NF, Zetoune FS, Sarma JV, et al. Extracellular histones are essential effectors of C5aR- and C5L2-mediated tissue damage and inflammation in acute lung injury. FASEB J. 2013;27(12):5010–21 Epub 2013/08/29.

68. Yokoyama TT, S.; Nishi, J.; Yamashita, Y.; Ichikado, K.; Gushima, Y.; Ando, M. Hyperoxia-induced acute lung injury using a pig model: coreelation between MR imaging and histolgic results. Radiat Med. 2001;19(3):131–43.

69. Chandra A, Lan S, Zhu J, Lin T, Zhang X, Siclari VA, et al. PTH prevents the adverse effects of focal radiation on bone architecture in young rats. Bone. 2013;55(2):449–57 Epub 2013/03/08.

70. Detombe SAD-B, J.; Petrov, I. E.; Drangova, M. X-ray dose delivered during a longitudinal micro-CT study has no adverse effect on cardiac and pulmonary tissue in C57Bl/6 mice. Acta Radiol. 2013;54(4):435–41.

71. Greschus S, Kiessling F, Lichy MP, Moll J, Mueller MM, Savai R, et al. Potential applications of flat-panel volumetric CT in morphologic, functional small animal imaging. Neoplasia. 2005;7(8):730–40.

72. McVerry BJ, Peng X, Hassoun PM, Sammani S, Simon BA, Garcia JG. Sphingosine 1-phosphate reduces vascular leak in murine and canine models of acute lung injury. Am J Respir Crit Care Med. 2004;170(9):987–93 Epub 2004/07/30.

73. Zhou Z, Kozlowski J, Schuster DP. Physiologic, biochemical, and imaging characterization of acute lung injury in mice. Am J Respir Crit Care Med. 2005;172(3):344–51 Epub 2005/05/17.

74. Shofer S, Badea C, Auerbach S, Schwartz DA, Johnson GA. A micro-computed tomography-based method for the measurement of pulmonary compliance in healthy and bleomycin-exposed mice. Exp Lung Res. 2007;33(3–4):169–83 Epub 2007/06/15.

75. Perchiazzi G, Rylander C, Derosa S, Pellegrini M, Pitagora L, Polieri D, et al. Regional distribution of lung compliance by image analysis of computed tomograms. Respir Physiol Neurobiol. 2014;201:60–70 Epub 2014/07/16.

76. Fernandez-Bustamante A, Easley RB, Fuld M, Mulreany D, Chon D, Lewis JF, et al. Regional pulmonary inflammation in an endotoxemic ovine acute lung injury model. Respir Physiol Neurobiol. 2012;183(2):149–58 Epub 2012/06/26.

77. Cereda M XY, Kadlecek S, Hamedani H, Rajaei J, Clapp J, Rizi R. Hyperpolarized gas diffusion MRI for the study of atelectasis and acute respiratory distress syndrome. 2014.

78. Mintun MD, DR; Welch, MJ; Mathias, CJ; Schuster, DP. Measurements of pulmonary vascular permeability with PET and gallium-68 transferrin. J Nucl Med. 1987;28:1704–16.

79. Zambelli V, Di Grigoli G, Scanziani M, Valtorta S, Amigoni M, Belloli S, et al. Time course of metabolic activity and cellular infiltration in a murine model of acid-induced lung injury. Intensive Care Med. 2012;38(4):694–701 Epub 2012/01/27.

80. Pouzot C, Richard JC, Gros A, Costes N, Lavenne F, Le Bars D, et al. Noninvasive quantitative assessment of pulmonary blood flow with 18F-FDG PET. J Nucl Med. 2013;54 (9):1653–60 Epub 2013/08/03.

81. Audi SH, Jacobs ER, Zhao M, Roerig DL, Haworth ST, Clough AV. In vivo detection of hyperoxia-induced pulmonary endothelial cell death using (99 m)Tc-duramycin. Nucl Med Biol. 2015;42(1):46–52 Epub 2014/09/15.

82. Max MN, B.; Dembinski, R.; Schulz, G.; Kuhlen, R.; Buell, U.; Rossaint, R. Changes in pulmonary blood flow during gaseous and partial liquid ventilation in experimental acute lung injury. Anesthesiology. 2000;96(6):1437–45.

83. Lamm WG, MM; Albert, RK. Mechanism by which the prone position improves oxygenation in acute lung injury. Am J Respir Crit Care Med. 1994;150:184–93.

84. Murugkar S, Smith B, Srivastava P, Moica A, Naji M, Brideau C, et al. Miniaturized multimodal CARS microscope based on MEMS scanning and a single laser source. Opt Express. 2010;18(23):23796–804 Epub 2010/12/18.

85. Chagnon F, Fournier C, Charette PG, Moleski L, Payet MD, Dobbs LG, et al. In vivo intravital endoscopic confocal fluorescence microscopy of normal and acutely injured rat lungs. Lab Invest J Tech Methods Pathol. 2010;90(6):824–34 Epub 2010/04/14.

86. Gu M, Kang H, Li X. Breaking the diffraction-limited resolution barrier in fiber-optical two-photon fluorescence endoscopy by an azimuthally-polarized beam. Sci Rep. 2014;4:3627 Epub 2014/01/11.

87. Dames C, Akyuz L, Reppe K, Tabeling C, Dietert K, Kershaw O, et al. Miniaturized bronchoscopy enables unilateral investigation, application, and sampling in mice. Am J Respir Cell Mol Biol. 2014;51(6):730–7 Epub 2014/06/25.

Chapter 9
Genetic and Genomic Approaches to Acute Lung Injury

Ivana V. Yang

Introduction to Acute Lung Injury

Acute lung injury (ALI) and acute respiratory distress syndrome (ARDS) refer to milder and more severe forms, respectively, of a critical illness syndrome with high mortality (38.5 %) and incidence estimates at 58.7–86.2/100,000 person-years [1]. Both forms of the disease are defined by hypoxemic respiratory failure that is characterized by severe impairment of gas exchange and lung mechanics with bilateral pulmonary infiltrates that are not attributed to left atrial hypertension [1, 2]. The most recent Berlin definition eliminated ALI as a clinical category and established mild, moderate, and severe categories of ARDS; however ALI is still used as a broad term for the clinical syndrome and in the research setting [2]. Substantial phenotypic heterogeneity underlies ALI [3]; for example, ALI caused by direct (pulmonary) and indirect (extrapulmonary) causes have a number of differences in clinical presentation and site of injury (epithelial vs endothelial).

The most common predisposing conditions for developing ALI are sepsis, pneumonia, and shock [2]. While demographic factors such as gender and race/ethnicity are not independent risk factors for ALI, they seem to affect mortality associated with this syndrome [2]. Age, on the other hand, is a strong risk factor for ALI with incidence increasing with age [2]. Similar to other complex lung diseases, development of ALI is influenced by both genetic and environmental factors. Genetic variation explains some of the heterogeneity in patients' risk for development of ALI

I.V. Yang (✉)
Department of Medicine, University of Colorado Anschutz Medical Campus, Aurora, USA
e-mail: Ivana.yang@ucdenver.edu

I.V. Yang
Department of Epidemiology, Colorado School of Public Health, Aurora, USA

I.V. Yang
Center for Genes, Environment, and Health, National Jewish Health, Denver, USA

© Springer International Publishing AG 2017
L.M. Schnapp and C. Feghali-Bostwick (eds.), *Acute Lung Injury and Repair*,
Respiratory Medicine, DOI 10.1007/978-3-319-46527-2_9

with genetic variants in >30 genes associated with ALI to date [4]. The strongest environmental risk factor for ALI is alcohol use followed by tobacco use and possibly air pollution [5] while diabetes appears to be protective, an association that is incompletely understood [6].

At the molecular level, ALI is characterized by inflammatory injury to the alveolar capillary barrier, with extravasation of protein-rich edema fluid into the airspace [7]. Systemic inflammation, defined by increase in pro-inflammatory cytokines (TNF-α, IL-1β, IL-6, and IL-8), is a hallmark of ALI and the innate immune system plays a crucial role in the initiation of the inflammatory cascade [7]. Toll-like receptors (TLRs) [8] and nucleotide-binding oligomerization domain-like receptors (NLRs) [9] on multiple cell types but especially monocytes/macrophages recognize exogenous and endogenous dangers, pathogen-associated molecular patterns (PAMPs) and damage-associated molecular patterns (DAMPs), respectively, and initiate the inflammatory cascade. Another important aspect of innate immunity is the training and tolerance that occur upon multiple challenges with microbial products. Macrophages/monocytes that are stimulated with β-glucan from *Candida albicans* (dectin-1 ligand) become more responsive upon restimulation, a demonstration of a priming effect or a state of trained immunity [10] which is thought to be important in the prevention of secondary infections. On the other hand, macrophages/monocytes treated with lipopolysaccharide (LPS; TLR4 ligand) become unresponsive upon restimulation (produce significantly lower concentrations of pro-inflammatory cytokines compared to cells that are only stimulated once). There is increasing evidence that macrophages/monocytes form patients with sepsis may be tolerized [11]. Neutrophils also play an important role in the pathophysiology of ALI. Neutrophil infiltration is an early step in the acute inflammatory response to tissue injury or infection and these cells are equipped with a variety of mechanisms to recognize and kill invading microbial pathogens and remove damaged cells [7, 12].

Given the genetic and environmental components of ALI, it is important to understand genetic variants, transcriptional profiles, and epigenetic marks in this disease. This Chapter will focus on study design for genome-wide level analysis of genetic variants, coding and noncoding RNAs, and epigenetic marks; methods for genomic analysis and focused approaches for validation of genomic hits and independent replication; and progress that has been made to date in ALI with specific focus on human studies. At the end of the Chapter, future directions and integrative analyses of these datasets, together with additional—omic data not discussed in this Chapter (microbiome, metabolome, proteome) will be discussed briefly.

General Design and Statistical Considerations for Genome-Wide Studies

The overall flow of how genome-wide studies are conducted is common to the three areas of discussion (Fig. 9.1). In each section, we will discuss genome-wide approaches and targeted techniques that can be used for both internal (technical)

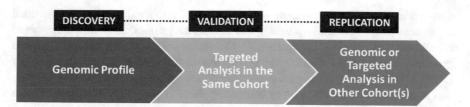

Fig. 9.1 Conceptual approach to overall study design for genomic assessment of genetic variants, transcriptome, and epigenetic marks in which internal (technical) and external (replication) validation are performed to ensure validity and generalizability of findings from the genomic analysis

and external (replication) validation. Technical validation of the findings from genome-wide scans is commonly performed by targeted approaches that will be discussed in each section. Similarly, replication of findings from the discovery phase of the study in independent cohort(s) is a gold standard with well-defined criteria in studies of genetic variants [13], has been done extensively in gene expression signature studies [14], and is becoming important in epigenetic studies [15, 16]. However, due to influence of both genetic and environmental factors on the epigenome, replication in these studies is a bit more complex than in genetic studies.

The most important consideration in the study design for any genome-wide study is power [17] to detect significant associations given the large number of tests that are performed in the analysis phase. Power depends greatly on the number of individuals in the cohort but also on the effects size which is directly related to the strength and homogeneity of the trait/clinical phenotype of interest. Unfortunately, many of the complex diseases including ALI are heterogeneous in nature and thus an important consideration in the study design phase is whether there is a more homogeneous clinical subphenotype that should be analyzed; this should be balanced with the cohort size. In addition to the trait/clinical phenotype of interest, demographic characteristics such as age, gender, and race/ethnicity need to be considered when designing a genome-wide study as they can be confounders in the analysis if not appropriately taken into account. When using next generation sequencing methods, sequence depth and coverage are additional important considerations for all genomic studies [18].

Statistical approaches for controlling for multiple comparisons are also common to the three areas of discussion in this Chapter. The most conservative approach is the Bonferroni correction in which case the p value is multiplied by the number of comparisons that are performed. The assumption for this method is that each association test is independent of all other tests, an assumption that is generally untrue in the biological setting as there are correlations in genetic variants, epigenetic marks, and gene expression across the genome. An alternative that is often used is the false discovery rate (FDR) correction, developed by Benjamini and Hochberg, in which case FDR correction is made for the number of expected false discoveries, providing an estimate of the number of true results among those called significant [19]. The final approach that is sometimes used is permutation-based adjustment for multiple comparisons. This computationally intensive approach generates an empirical distribution of the test statistic based on a large number (1000 or more) random assignments of the phenotype to the genome-wide profile that is used to asses significance by comparing minimal p value from the real data to that distribution [17].

Genome

The human genome sequence provides the underlying code for human biology. Our genome is composed of 3 billion base pairs and about 20,687 protein-coding genes. Protein-coding regions comprise 1.2 % of the genome and are referred to as the exome (collection of exons). The remainder of the genome is involved in regulation of the protein-coding genes [20–22]. Variations in the DNA sequence are important susceptibility factors for complex common diseases and syndromes such as ALI.

Common Variants

The main focus of complex disease genetics for the past 10–15 years has been the identification of common genetic risk variants (allele frequencies >5 %) [23]. The basis for this search is the Common Disease Common Variant (CDCV) hypothesis, which assumes that a relatively small number of ancient common risk alleles exist that each confer small to moderate risks of disease. The CDCV hypothesis was testable in this timeframe in a number of complex diseases due to several practical considerations: [1] the high frequency of putative risk alleles, allowing for cost-effective analysis by genotyping as opposed to sequencing; [2] the extensive linkage disequilibrium (LD, correlation) [24] between common variants in the human genome, which allows for genotyping only a small number of markers (LD tags) and indirect assessment of other common variants by LD mapping; and [3] the development of high-throughput genotyping arrays, which have allowed Genome-Wide Association (GWA) studies. Consequently more than 2000 GWA studies exploring the role of common variants in several hundred complex diseases or phenotypes have been conducted to date [25].

Study Design

GWA study can be of a case-control design of unrelated individuals with the disease phenotype of interest (cases) and unaffected individuals (controls) or of a quantitative phenotype [26]. The key feature of these studies is that they are based on association analysis and therefore require unrelated individuals (as opposed to genetic linkage studies in which families are required).

Technologies

Dense genotyping arrays containing hundreds of thousands to millions of markers have been developed for GWA studies. Two major commercial sources of geno-typing arrays are Illumina and Affymetrix and they offer a variety of specific array platforms that should be chosen based on study population and hypothesis of the project. Selection of markers that are included on the genotyping arrays has relied largely of HapMap [27] and more recently 1000 Genome [28] projects. Specific content has been developed to provide a variety of array platforms that range from basic coverage to make large-scale projects affordable (OmniExpress Bead Chip, for example) to providing the most comprehensive coverage across multiple populations (Omni2.5 Bead Chip for example that was designed using 1000 Genome data).

Analysis

Analysis of common genetic variants is performed in three steps: [1] testing for departures from Hardy–Weinberg Equilibrium (HWE) proportions; [2] estimate of variant–variant LD to assess the genetic structure of the cohort [24]; and [3] association analysis under a specific genetic model (additive, recessive, or dominant) via logistic regression. Logistic regression models usually include demographic covariates such as age and gender. Instead of using basic race/ethnicity categories from self-reports, principal components (PCs) from the genome-wide genetic variant data are also included in the regression model. This is done because even among a sample of a single racial/ethnic group such as nonhispanic white individuals, consideration of the effects of population stratification is very important. Significance level in GWA studies is most commonly assessed using the concept of genome-wide significance, which uses an estimated number of independent genomic regions based on the distribution of LD in the genome for a specific population; for European populations, this is approximately $p < 5 \times 10^{-8}$ [17].

One of the fundamental concepts in the analysis of GWA studies is that of meta-analysis. In this approach, findings from multiple studies can be combined to increase the power of identification of significant genetic variants. An essential principle in meta-analysis is that all studies included examined the same hypothesis and that the original analysis was performed in an almost identical fashion [29]; when this is not possible, statistical approaches to assess heterogeneity of analysis methods are used [26]. Software package METAL is often used for meta-analysis of GWA studies [30] and detailed protocols for this type of study have been published [31].

Imputation analysis of genotype data is often performed in GWA studies for two reasons: [1] to identify additional genetic risk loci, and [2] to provide information on the same set of variants and thus facilitate meta-analysis. In this approach, a reference panel such as Hapmap or 1000 Genome data are used in conjunction with genotype data to infer genotypes that were not directly measured on the genotyping array using haplotypes (groups of variants that are inherited together, or are in high LD, in a specific population). The most important consideration in imputation is to use the reference population that is best matched to the study cohort. In practice, study sample haplotypes may match multiple reference haplotype and imputation assigns probability of the presence of specific allele(s). This analysis is performed using software such as IMPUTE [32] or MaCH [33].

While tools for functional annotation of genetic variants can be applied to most significant hits from the GWAS analysis, additional fine mapping by denser genotyping or sequencing is generally required to identify variants that are likely to have functional consequences. Functional annotation strategies are discussed in the next section.

Rare Genetic Variants

While GWA studies have provided a wealth of information on the genetic basis of common complex diseases, they have generally explained a small portion of disease heritability even after judiciously designed GWA studies screening >1 million markers in large groups of cases and controls have been carried out. The "missing heritability" problem has elicited interest in the potential role of rare variants in complex disease. Under the Common Disease Rare Variant (CDRV) hypothesis, any given risk gene or locus is characterized by high allelic heterogeneity and these risk loci contain multiple rare independent risk alleles across the population each with moderate to high penetrance. As a consequence of expected allelic heterogeneity, sequencing rather than genotyping is required for exploration of the CDRV hypothesis in complex diseases. Furthermore, screening of these rare alleles is not amenable to LD tagging approaches as they are poorly tagged by common variants and individual rare variants are expected to occur on different haplotypes (a group of variants that are inherited together). The emergence of massively parallel sequencing technologies has dramatically reduced the time and cost of study population sequencing, setting the stage for exploration of the CDRV hypothesis in complex diseases. Different models of the genetic basis of complex traits are discussed in detail elsewhere [34].

Study Design

Whole genome, whole exome, and targeted sequencing projects are mostly designed to identify rare genetic variants but they will also capture information on common variation. Whole genome sequencing (WGS) studies capture variation in both coding and noncoding variants while whole exome sequencing (WES) studies are focused on coding variants (although newer target enrichment strategies capture UTRs and some promoter and intronic sequence). WES is ∼10 fold less expensive than WGS thus allowing for a larger number of samples to be profiled, and the data produced are less complex to analyze. Targeted resequencing studies are well suited for following up on GWAS or linkage loci and are generally designed to capture the entire locus, including both coding and noncoding regions. Loci with previously associated common variants through GWAS can be fine mapped and are more likely to contain functional rare variants and therefore may be the most fruitful application of next generation sequencing to complex disease. It was initially proposed that two affordable strategies for identification of disease-causing variants were [1] sequencing of affected individuals in a pedigree followed by genotyping of candidate variants to demonstrate co-segregation with disease in the family and [2] extreme-trait sequencing of a small number of individuals at the tails of the trait distribution followed by targeted sequencing or genotyping in a larger cohort [35, 36]. As the cost of sequencing has decreased, other study designs have been adopted. Statistical considerations for the design of rare variant association studies are discussed in detail elsewhere [37].

Technologies

The first sequences of the human genome published a decade ago [38, 39] were accomplished using automated Sanger sequencing with dideoxy chain termination [40] at a cost of approximately $2.7 billion to produce a draft sequence of the human genome (http://www.genome.gov/11006943). In contrast, today a human genome can be sequenced at $20\times$ coverage for roughly $2500 using next generation sequencing (NGS) technology. NGS refers to a group of strategies that rely on a combination of template preparation, sequencing and imaging, and genome alignment and assembly methods, producing gigabases (GB) of sequence data per run in the form of short reads [41]. The Illumina sequencing platform is the most commonly used at the present time and its read length is currently capped at 2×125 bp. Single molecule technologies such as from Pacific Biosciences do not require the clonal amplification of molecules to be sequenced, but rather a single DNA molecule is sequenced by synthesis using a DNA polymerase. Single molecule sequencing technologies promise a much simpler sample preparation and offer longer read lengths but generally have lower accuracy than short-read sequencers, which makes them less desirable for rare variant studies. However, their long read lengths are useful in the regions of the genome that are difficult to assemble using short reads, with highly repetitive genomic regions being the best example. A combination of short and long read length technologies provides the best solution in some cases. Single molecule technology is reviewed elsewhere [42].

Another important aspect of sequencing exomes or genomic regions of interest, such as those identified by GWA studies, is target capture. Large genomic regions are most efficiently and cost-effectively captured using hybridization-based approaches such as Agilent SureSelect and Nimblegen SeqCap while PCR-based approaches offered by Life Technologies AmpliSeq and Agilent Haloplex are more suited for capture of smaller regions [43].

Analysis

Four main steps in the analysis of sequencing data are [1] base calling and sequence assembly [2], variant detection [3], statistical analysis to identify significant associations, and [4] functional analysis of the identified variants. Several recent reviews have detailed discussion of these steps [36, 44, 45] with the most important points briefly summarized here. Data analysis workflow begins with the base calling and alignment of sequence data to the reference genome [46]. Base-calling procedures generate per-base quality values (QVs) that are typically converted to Phred-like quality score [47]. Most alignment software provides run metrics that allow the user to assess quality of sequence data; these include number of raw reads, number of mapped reads, number of unique reads, sequence coverage, and coverage for and percent of "on target" reads for targeted approached [44]. The quality controls metrics allow the researchers to determine potential experimental and alignment biases and remove low quality and poorly mapping reads from further analysis.

The high quality, aligned reads are then analyzed to identify DNA sequence variants, most commonly single nucleotide variants (SNVs); information on structural variants (SVs) and copy number variants (CNVs) can also be obtained. Multiple software options exist for variant calling with both those that perform variant calls in individual samples and those that use multiple samples to call variants [45, 47]; commonly used pipelines include GATK [48] and SAMTools [49], among others. Single marker statistical analysis of common variants (>5 % MAF) from sequence data is identical to that used for GWA studies. On the other hand, most study populations will be underpowered to conduct single marker tests of association for rare variants (0.1–1 % range of MAF) despite the expectation of high effect sizes for rare risk alleles (relative risks ~ 2.5–5.0). The general approach taken is therefore to test for association between disease status and the accumulation of rare variants across the risk locus or gene units rather than with any single variant. Three main classes of collapsing tests are [1] tests that use group summary statistics on variant frequencies in cases and controls; [2] those that test for similarity in unique DNA sequences in different individuals; and [3] regression models that test collapsed sets of variants (and other variables) as predictors of the phenotype [36]. Many of the features of the different approaches are combined in a single software SKAT-O, where O refers to optimal [50] that is commonly used in these analyses.

Following association testing, identified variants are analyzed for functional consequences. Algorithms that predict deleteriousness of protein-coding variants such as SIFT or PolyPhen are used to prioritize nonsense and frameshift mutations because they result in loss of protein function [51, 52]. SIFT has been incorporated into ANNOVAR pipeline [53] while PolyPhen is a part of the SeattleSeq pipeline (http://snp.gs.washington.edu/SeattleSeqAnnotation) as well as the PLINK/SEQ suite (http://atgu.mgh.harvard.edu/plinkseq/) for comprehensive functional annotation of variants. Methods for prioritizing noncoding variants based on nucleotide sequence conservation are also being utilized in large-scale sequencing studies; one commonly used of the many available algorithms (listed in Ref. [54]) is the Genomic Evolutionary Rate Profiling (GERP) algorithm [55]. These algorithms use comparative genomics, generally limited to mammalian species as nucleotide sequence is less conserved than protein sequence, to estimate nucleotide-level evolutionary constraints in genomic sequence alignments and assign conservation scores. Higher conservation scores are indicative of a more likely regulatory function and can be used to prioritize noncoding variants for further studies. A recently developed Combined Annotation–Dependent Depletion (CADD) method integrates many diverse measures of functional relevance such as deleteriousness, conservation, and other scored into a single measure (C score) for each variant that can be used to objectively prioritize variants [56]. An alternative to post hoc analysis of variants in associated genes/loci is to incorporate functional information into the test and stratify or weigh rare alleles by functional significance. A number of tests allow for inclusion of prediction scores in test statistics; PLINK/SEQ, for example, includes previously computed PolyPhen scores [57].

Targeted Methods for Validation

The choice of the platform for internal or technical validation of variants identified by genome-wide technologies is guided by the frequency of the variant and number of samples. The most cost-effective way to validate variants with low frequencies is usually to directly sequence the region that contains multiple rare variants in different individuals. This is achieved by Sanger sequencing or PCR-based next generation strategies such as the IonTorrent Ampliseq platform. On the other hand, variants with higher frequencies can be genotyped at a lower cost than sequencing using targeted genotyping panels; Illumina, Sequenom, and Fluidigm, to name a few, have solutions for custom genotyping panels.

Progress to Date in ALI

Because of the nature of ALI, specifically the fact that it does not occur spontaneously but as an outcome of severe illness, no family pedigrees exist and therefore early linkage studies that identified some regions of the genome of interest in other lung diseases such as asthma could not be performed in ALI. Despite this, it is thought that genetic factors influence individual's predisposition to development of severe illness, ALI/ARDS, and response to treatment in a multistage genetic risk model that has been proposed [4]. This is further supported by the established role of genetic variation in the control of host response to stimulation with PAMPs and other innate immune stimuli [58–60].

Early studies of association of SNPs in candidate genes in inflammatory and other relevant pathways with ALI phenotypes are summarized in [61]. More recent candidate gene studies have identified association of SNPs in the elafin or peptidase inhibitor 3 (*PI3*) gene with increased risk of ARDS [62], *ANGPT2* genetic variant with trauma-associated ALI [63], *IL1RN* coding variant with lower risk of ARDS [64] as well as SNPs in an adiponectin-like gene *ADIPOQ* [65] and colony stimulating factor 2 (*CSF2*) [66] with higher mortality, among others. Because of the prominent role of platelet levels in the pathophysiology of ALI/ARDS, another targeted study examined association of genetic variants in five loci previously associated with platelet levels through a meta-analysis with ARDS outcomes. This work confirmed the importance of *LRRC16A* in platelet formation and suggested a role for it in ARDS pathophysiology [67]. Importantly, distinct genetic risk factors have been identified as associated with ARDS caused by direct versus indirect injury to the lung [68], demonstrating that study of more homogeneous clinical phenotypes is critical in genetic studies.

Genomic assessments of the effect of genetic variants of ALI phenotypes are just emerging. The first GWAS of 600 ALI cases and 2266 controls followed by replication in 212 cases and 283 controls identified 159 significant SNPs ($p < 0.05$ for replication) associated with risk of ALI, providing support for further evaluation of genetic variation in this syndrome. Similarly, an exome sequencing study of 96 ARDS cases compared to 1000 Genome control data identified 89 SNPs associated with susceptibility to ARDS, with a few of these variants also associated with severity as assessed by the APACHE II score as well as mortality [62].

Transcriptome

The transcriptome is the collection of all the RNA molecules, or transcripts, present in a cell. DNA is transcribed by RNA polymerase to create complementary RNA strands, which in turn are spliced to remove introns, producing mature transcripts that contain only exons, which are translated into protein. While only a small percentage of the human transcriptome is translated into proteins, a number of proteins have different isoforms that stem from alternatively spliced transcripts. The remaining transcriptome is largely comprised of a number of noncoding RNAs that are involved in regulation of gene expression; these include thousands of pseudo-genes [69], circular RNAs [70], long noncoding RNAs [71], and small noncoding RNAs [71]. The most well studied group of noncoding RNAs are microRNAs (miRNAs). They control gene expression by binding to the 3′ untranslated regions (UTRs) of messenger RNA (mRNA), which leads to either mRNA degradation or inhibition of protein translation. Regulation of gene expression by miRNAs is complex in that many miRNAs can regulate expression of a single gene and, similarly, each miRNA can regulate a large number of genes. Other noncoding RNAs are reviewed in detail elsewhere [71].

Study Design

Study design for genome-wide assessment of coding and noncoding RNA is in principle the same with two important considerations: power to detect association with the outcome variable of interest, and potential confounders including covariates and batch effects. Power and covariates were discussed in the general design section. Batch effects are broadly classified as known (amount of labeled RNA, date of library preparation or hybridization, position on the array, lane on the sequencing run, etc.) and unknown batch effects. While statistical approaches for correcting for known and unknown batch effects are available and will be discussed in the analysis section, care should be taken during study design to minimize the effect of known batch effects. This is done by assigning samples from each experimental group to each set or batch of labeling reactions, library preparation, hybridization, sequencing lane, etc., for small sample sizes or randomizing across batches for larger sample sizes [72].

Technologies

Genomic profiling of gene expression levels in lung disease began as early as in other diseases and used both homemade cDNA arrays and some of the first commercially available arrays that both suffered from many technical issues [73–75]. However, substantial improvements in both laboratory and analytical aspects of microarray-based analysis of gene expression have occurred [76, 77] and genomic analysis of gene expression on microarrays has reached maturity to become a fairly standard approach. Major providers of gene expression arrays are Affymetrix, Agilent, and Illumina and they all use one-color assays at this time (some of the older platforms used two colors).

RNA sequencing-based approaches were introduced much more recently and are not as mature as microarrays [78]. While protocols for library preparation and sequencing are fairly standard at this time, best practices for data analysis of RNA-seq data are still under development (and will be discussed in the next section). Sequencing of polyA-enriched libraries at relatively low coverage is the most affordable form of RNA-seq and gives information on coding transcripts that is comparable to microarrays. Sequencing of the same library at higher coverage results in an expanded detection limit for more rare transcripts and data can also be analyzed for alternative splicing. On the other hand, sequencing of ribosomal RNA-depleted libraries provides information on coding and noncoding RNAs. One extension of this protocol is dual RNA-seq for capturing transcriptome information on both the host and pathogens [79]. Small RNA-seq library preparation protocols are required to capture mature small RNA species such as miRNAs. An important note is that standard RNA extraction protocols do not always capture small RNA and therefore care must be taken in this step to capture them if they are of interest to the study.

The most exciting advance in RNA-seq technology in the past few years has been the extension to single cell analysis of the transcriptome. In this approach, technologies such as that offered by Fluidigm are used to isolate single cells, often following flow cytometry or other methods for selection of pure cell populations, and create cDNA in 96-well plate format that can be used for either standard quantitative PCR or RNA-seq library preparation. While the cost of this type of experiment is high due to the need to sequence large numbers of single cells, it is somewhat offset by the fact that lower sequencing coverage is needed for single cells. This technology has recently been used to provide a greater molecular understanding of lung development and cell lineages in the lung [80] and is a promising approach to understand molecular underpinnings of lung diseases such as ALI.

Analysis

The main steps in the analysis of transcriptome data are: [1] alignment of sequence data in the case of RNA-seq [2] normalization and scaling [3], assessment of batch effects, and [4] identification of differentially expressed genes or noncoding RNAs. The output of a microarray experiment is background-subtracted set of intensities for all probes on the array. The output of RNA-seq data are short read sequences that first need to be aligned to the genome with gapped sequence aligners such as TopHat [81] and quantified relative to known genes in the genome using software such as BEDTools [82]. More detailed consideration of sequence alignment and read quantification for transcriptome analysis is presented in [83, 84]. Both array and RNA-seq data need to be normalized and scaled so that across-sample comparisons can be made. The most commonly used normalization approach is quantile normalization such as robust multi-array average (RMA) [85] or similar approaches tailored for RNA-seq data [86].

The effect of known batch effects can be examined using correlation to top principal components to identify confounding variables that explain a significant portion of variation in the dataset [72]; these variables can then be included downstream in the statistical analysis. Unknown batch effects can also be dealt with by estimating latent variables that explain observed variation in the data that are not due to variables of interest. This is a more complex approach that requires a deeper understanding of the statistics but implementations such as surrogate value analysis (SVA) [87] and probabilistic estimation of expression residuals (PEER) [88] have been developed for this purpose. Prior to statistical analysis, array intensities or RNA-seq counts are log2-transformed and sometimes filters are applied to remove genes that do not vary across all samples with the goal of reducing the multiple testing burden [89].

The choice of the statistical model for identification of differentially expressed transcripts or noncoding RNAs depends on the experimental design. Simple t-test is used for two-group comparison in cases where adjustment for additional covariates is not needed. In order of increasing complexity, other models that are used are analysis of (co)variance [AN(C)OVA] or linear models for inclusion of more than two groups and adjustment for covariates, repeated-measures, and mixed-effects linear models. The most commonly used software package for analysis of array data is limma as it allows for use of moderated t-statistic [90]. Statistical analysis of RNA-seq data is still evolving as methods that have been developed for microarray data are not ideal due to the discrete nature of RNA-Seq data. Negative binomial distribution is most often used in the analysis of count data as it accounts for overdispersion (variance > mean) with several implementations including DESeq [91] and EdgeR [92] that are commonly used. Complexities and challenges involved in the analysis of RNA-seq data are discussed in detail in [93]. Discussion of alternate transcript use analysis, using software such as Cufflinks [94], and specialized approaches for dual RNA-seq [79] and single cell RNA-seq analysis [95] is beyond the scope of this overview chapter.

Targeted Methods for Validation

Validation of genes or noncoding RNAs that are identified as statistically significant by microarray or RNA-seq can be accomplished using several approaches with the most cost- and time-effective approach depending on the number of samples and number of RNAs to be validated. Most methods rely on quantitative real-time PCR, using Taqman or SYBRGreen as detection strategies. Basic qPCR performed in either 96- or 384-well format is a standard approach in most laboratories but there are also more mid- to high-throughput approaches such as Fluidigm, SABiosciences, and Life Technologies TLDA and OpenArray. Another newer technology that is gaining popularity as it is fairly high-throughput and has high sensitivity is the NanoString nCounter technology. Regardless of the specific technology, these assays are generally performed in triplicate for accuracy and require a parallel analysis of housekeeping gene(s). Data from qPCR assays are most often analyzed using the $\Delta\Delta Ct$ relative expression analysis [96] but there are cases in which a standard curve approach to be able to report absolute number of copies of the RNA is warranted.

Progress to Date in ALI

Transcriptional profiles of human monocyte response to innate immune stimuli have been studied extensively [97] as have been contributions of miRNAs [98] to regulation of gene expression while the role of long noncoding RNAs is also emerging [99]. Microarray profiling of gene expression in alveolar macrophages and circulating leukocytes in different patient populations has demonstrated the importance of the inflammasome [100] and neutrophil-related genes [101], and identified biomarkers of disease [101–103], among others [104]. RNA-seq technology is only beginning to be used is studies of ALI [105] and holds a great promise for providing a deeper understanding of coding and noncoding RNAs in the pathogenesis of this syndrome. Expression of miRNAs, for example, has only been examined using microarrays in animal models but not in human cohorts [106].

Epigenome

Much of the 80 % of the genome sequence that is predicted to be regulatory includes promoter, enhancer, insulator, and other elements throughout the genome [22, 107] that are labeled by epigenetic marks. Epigenetic processes translate environmental exposures into regulation of chromatin, which shapes the identity, gene expression profile, and activity of specific cell types that participate in disease pathophysiology [108]. Two main classes of epigenetic marks are DNA methylation and modifications of histone tails, although noncoding RNAs are sometimes considered a part of the epigenome.

DNA Methylation

Methylation of cytosine residues in CpG dinucleotides (5-methylcytosine) in CpG islands is the simplest form of epigenetic regulation with hypermethylation of CpG islands in gene promoters leading to gene silencing and hypomethylation leading to active transcription [109, 110]. It has been more recently demonstrated that methylation of less CpG dense regions near islands ("CpG island shores") [111, 112] and within gene bodies [113, 114] is also important in regulation of gene transcription and alternative splicing and that the relationship between methylation and transcription is much more complex than the canonical inverse relationship. Further adding to this complexity is the presence of methylation marks in non-CpG context in embryonic stem cells [115] and the presence of 5-hydroxymethylcytosine, which may be a mark of demethylation [116]. DNA methyltransferases (de novo DNMT3A/B and maintenance DNMT1) are enzymes responsible for DNA methylation while the TET family of enzymes actively demethylates DNA through the 5-hydoxymethylcytosine intermediate [116].

Study Design

Study design for epigenome-wide association studies (EWAS) of DNA methylation follows many of the same basic principles for the genomic studies of DNA variants and the transcriptome and is discussed in detail in recent review articles [15, 16]. In addition to sample size, phenotype heterogeneity, and potential confounders (covariates and batch effects), two additional criteria that are considered in determining power of an EWAS are whether tissues/cells are those from the target organ or a surrogate and how pure the cell population is. The ideal situation for the study of DNA methylation would be to have a fairly pure cell population of interest from the lung. This, however, is difficult to achieve in human cohort studies so surrogate cells, defined as nontarget readily accessible cell types, are often used in epigenetic studies. While more work needs to be done to identify best surrogate cells for DNA methylation studies, in general the signal is lower in surrogate than target cells requiring larger sample sizes. Similarly, epigenetic marks are cell specific and the more pure the cell population is the stronger the signal will be; if a mixture of cells is profiled, a larger sample size will be required. Another complication of using mixed cell populations is that systematic bias in cell population composition between the groups being tested can result in DNA methylation changes due to differences in cell composition rather than altered epigenetic patterns within each cell type associated with the disease.

Technologies

Microarrays have been the method of choice for profiling epigenetic marks on a genomic scale, with several platforms and protocols available for DNA methylation— bisulfate conversion of methylated cytosines, methylated DNA immunoprecipitation (MeDIP) using an anti-methylcytosine antibody, and digestion of DNA with restriction enzymes specific for methylated or unmethylated cytosines [117]. The Illumina 450 k and the latest 850 k are the most commonly used platform for genomic analysis of DNA methylation in human cohorts at the present time. This array platfrom provides comprehensive coverage for 99 % of Refseq genes with 20 probes per gene on average covering both promoter and gene body. It simultaneously provides coverage for all CpG islands in the genome (five probes on average), CpG island shores (five probes on average), and more distant CpG motifs CpG shelves (four probes on average). More comprehensive sequencing-based approaches for the most informative areas of the genome for DNA methylation analysis are also beginning to be applied to human cohorts; these include Agilent SureSelect Methyl-seq [118] and Nimblegen SeqCAP Epi [119] target enrichment protocols. Whole genome bisulfite sequencing techniques have not been widely used in human cohorts due to the expense and the complexity involved in the analysis of such large datasets. Approaches for single-cell bisulfite sequencing are just emerging [120] and hold great promise for understanding the heterogeneity in epigenetic regulation of gene expression.

Another important aspect of DNA methylation studies is the ability to capture information on 5-hydroxymethylcytosine, a mark of demethylation. Bisulfite conversion captures both 5-methyl- and 5-hydroxymethylcytosine but methods that distinguish the two are reaching maturity and can be used in conjunction with the Illumina 450 k array [121] or sequencing [122, 123]. It should be noted, however, that two arrays or two sequencing runs are needed per sample to assess the relative contribution of 5-methyl- and 5-hydroxymethylcytosine.

Analysis

Methods that have been developed for the normalization of expression array data are not directly applicable to methylation array data due to bimodal distribution of percent methylation (beta value on the Illumina array). Transformation of beta to M values leads a more normal distribution and is commonly used but specialized approaches for analysis of methylation data are still required. Normalization is generally performed using a subset of probes on the array and approaches such as Subset-quantile Within Array Normalization (SWAN) also deal efficiently with normalization of two different types of probes present on the 450 k array [124]. Normalized data are subject to standard statistical models, as described in the transcriptome section, and adjustment for multiple comparisons. In addition to identification of statistically significant single CpG sites (differentially methylated positions or DMPs), approaches for identification of significant regions (differentially methylated regions or DMRs) [125, 126] can also be applied to Illumina data although they are more commonly used in the analysis of methylation sequencing data. An additional consideration in the analysis of Illumina array data is filtering of probes that contain SNPs as it is known that SNPs can affect binding and result in spurious methylation measurements [127]. Finally, while the best approach for adjustment for differences in cell composition is to use cell counts obtained independently, cell proportions in each sample can be estimated using methylation data and a reference dataset such as that available for peripheral blood cells [128] or a reference-free approach [129].

Targeted Methods for Validation

Validation of DNA methylation changes identified using genomic analysis requires techniques that are highly quantitative such as pyrosequencing [130] on the Qiagen Pyromark instruments and Epityper assays [131] on the Sequenom MassARRAY; both techniques can reliably detect methylation differences as small as 5 %. A comparison of the Illumina 450 k array and quantitative pyrosequencing revealed high concordance of percent methylation values on the two platforms [132].

Histone Modifications

Histones are proteins that enable DNA molecules to be tightly packaged into chromosomes inside the cell nucleus. While a number of different modifications exist, acetylation and methylation are the most common modifications of histone tails that occur at specific sites and residues, and control gene expression by regulating DNA accessibility to RNA polymerase II and transcription factors. Histone acetyltransferases (HATs) acetylate histone tails, histone deacetylases (HDACs) remove acetyl groups from histone tails, and bromodomain (Brd) proteins are chromatin readers that recognize and bind acetylated histones and play a key role in transmission of epigenetic memory across cell divisions and transcription regulation [133, 134]. Similarly, histone methyltransferases (HMTs) add the methyl groups to histone tails while histone demethylases (HDMs) remove them [133, 134]. Acetylation of lysine 27 on the histone H3 (H3K27ac) is, for example, one of the most informative single histone modifications. It is known to mark active enhancers and promoters [135].

Study Design

Study design for genomic assessment of histone modifications needs to take into account factors that have been discussed in previous sections, namely power considerations related to the number of samples per group, phenotype heterogeneity, potential confounders (covariates and batch effects), and sequence depth coverage. All studies of histone modifications rely on chromatin immunoprecipitation (ChIP) and another important consideration is inclusion of appropriate controls for ChIP experiments; these most commonly include DNA isolated from cells that have been cross-linked and fragmented under the same conditions as the immunoprecipitated DNA (input DNA), and a "mock" ChIP reaction with a control antibody (IgG control) [136, 137].

Technologies

While arrays have been used in the past for assessment of histone modifications, this ChIP-CHIp technology is obsolete at this time and next generation sequencing approach ChIP-seq is utilized almost exclusively. A crucial factor for success of ChIP-seq experiments is the quality of the antibody used as not all antibodies that are marketed as "ChIP grade" are appropriate for this application [136, 137]. The best strategy for selection of ChIP antibodies for histone marks is to use those that have been validated by ENCODE [107] and Roadmap Epigenomics [22]. Library preparation and sequencing of DNA following ChIP is a fairly standard protocol with recent advances in the use of small cell numbers [138, 139] and extensions of the technology to encompass additional techniques for understanding chromatin structure [140].

Analysis

Following sequence alignment and mapping to the genome, regions of ChIP enrichment are identified using software specifically designed for this purpose

[140]; one commonly used package is Model-based Analysis of ChIP-Seq (MACS) [141]. The output of these algorithms generally ranks called regions by absolute signal (read number) or by computed significance of enrichment (*p*-values). Differential enrichment across experimental groups can be identified using software used for analysis of RNA-seq data [140].

Targeted Methods for Validation

Targeted validation of genomic ChIP-seq hits is especially important given that ChIP-seq is much less quantitative in nature than techniques for the analysis of the transcriptome and DNA methylation. ChIP followed by qPCR on the DNA is the method of choice for quantitative assessment of histone modifications at specific genomic loci. The same controls (input and IgG) that are used in ChIP-seq are important to include in qPCR experiments as the enrichment of the histone modification at the locus is calculated relative to input DNA and specificity is assessed by comparison to the IgG control.

Progress to Date in ALI

While no studies to date have assessed the contribution of epigenetic marks on ALI phenotypes in human cohorts, there is extensive evidence for the role of this level of regulation of gene expression in innate immunity [142, 143]. Epigenetic marks, including both DNA methylation and histone modifications, in concert with transcription factors, determine the fate of undifferentiated myeloid cells towards different lineages [144]. Histone modification has also emerged as crucial regulator of innate immune memory and tolerance in monocytes/macrophages [144]. The seminal study in this area demonstrated that histone modifications regulate the gene expression in tolerized macrophages so that pro-inflammatory genes are repressed while antimicrobial genes continue to be expressed in LPS-tolerized cells [145]. A more recent study comprehensively characterized genomic profiles of macrophages that are primed by exposure to β-glucan or tolerized by exposure to LPS [146], by profiling histone marks at promoters (H3K4me3), distal regulatory elements (H3K4me1), and the active forms of both promoters and enhancers (H3K27ac) and combining with RNA-seq and DNase I-seq (chromatin accessibility) data, and identified changes in immune and metabolic pathways that are specific to undifferentiated, differentiated, primed, and tolerized cell state. Another study showed that histone modifications regulate the metabolic basis of trained immunity through induction of aerobic glycolysis through an Akt-mTOR-HIF-1α pathway [147]. These studies provide a foundation for the study of epigenetic regulation of gene expression in ALI.

Future Directions and Systems Biology

ALI is a complex heterogeneous disorder influenced by both genetics and environment. While genetic, transcriptomic, and epigenetic profiles have been understudied in relation to specific ALI phenotypes in human cohorts, omic studies of the innate immune response in cells and model organisms have been done and provide a good first step in understanding genetic and environmental influences on this syndrome. Once more individual datasets become available, the main challenge in ALI will be to understand how these different elements of the genome, transcriptome, and epigenome interact to ultimately lead to specific disease phenotypes.

Systems biology generally refers to a process of identifying networks of molecular pathways based on the evidence from the genome, transcriptome, and epigenome, as well as other -omic studies including the microbiome, proteome, and metabolome (Fig. 9.2). One of the key steps in understanding the genetic and environmental basis of ALI and identifying key targets for diagnostics and therapeutics will be sophisticated integrative systems-biology-level analysis of -omic

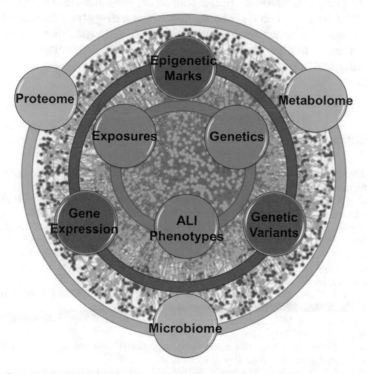

Fig. 9.2 Conceptual approach to systems biology analysis in ALI. Sophisticated network approaches will be required to integrate genomic datasets discussed in this Chapter (genome, transcriptome, and epigenome; *red*) with other—omic datasets (proteome, metabolome, microbiome; *green*) to understand the interplay between genetics and environment that leads to ALI clinical presentation (*blue*)

datasets [44, 148]. Some of the examples of integrative approaches are expression quantitative trait locus (eQTL) and methylation quantitative locus (meQTL) studies, which identify genetic variants or methylation marks that control gene expression levels [149, 150]. Other approaches rely on pathway analysis [151] of single datasets but can also be used for integration of multiple datasets. Pathway analyses are most often performed on the set of candidate genes from the genomic study using commercial approaches such as Ingenuity Pathway Analysis (IPA) [152] with its manually curated, weekly updated, and the largest knowledge base of its kind or noncommercial tools that incorporate network topology such as Signaling Pathway Impact Analysis (SPIA) [153] with its superior statistical approach for combining enrichment analysis and perturbation to the pathway (global pathway significance p value is calculated by combining enrichment and perturbation p-values). Other commonly used approaches include co-expression network analysis using Weighted Gene Correlation Network Analysis (WGCNA) [154] or testing for statistical significance of predefined sets of genes rather than single genes using approaches such as Gene Set Enrichment Analysis (GSEA) [155]. An additional level of integration is provided when rich publicly available datasets such as those collected by the ENCODE [107] and Roadmap Epigenomics [22] consortia are considered. Much more work is needed in refining these approaches as well applying them in a sensible fashion to complex diseases/syndromes such as ALI. Despite these challenges, a deeper understanding of genetic and environmental underpinnings of ALI will undoubtedly lead to better and more personalized therapeutic options for this deadly syndrome.

References

1. Rubenfeld GD, Caldwell E, Peabody E, Weaver J, Martin DP, Neff M, et al. Incidence and outcomes of acute lung injury. N Engl J Med. 2005;353(16):1685–93.
2. Sweatt AJ, Levitt JE. Evolving epidemiology and definitions of the acute respiratory distress syndrome and early acute lung injury. Clin Chest Med. 2014;35(4):609–24.
3. Reilly JP, Bellamy S, Shashaty MG, Gallop R, Meyer NJ, Lanken PN, et al. Heterogeneous phenotypes of acute respiratory distress syndrome after major trauma. Ann Am Thorac Soc. 2014;11(5):728–36.
4. Meyer NJ, Christie JD. Genetic heterogeneity and risk of acute respiratory distress syndrome. Semin Respir Crit Care Med. 2013;34(4):459–74.
5. Moazed F, Calfee CS. Environmental risk factors for acute respiratory distress syndrome. Clin Chest Med. 2014;35(4):625–37.
6. Honiden S, Gong MN. Diabetes, insulin, and development of acute lung injury. Crit Care Med. 2009;37(8):2455–64.
7. Han S, Mallampalli RK. The acute respiratory distress syndrome: from mechanism to translation. J Immunol. 2015;194(3):855–60.
8. O'Neill LA, Bowie AG. The family of five: TIR-domain-containing adaptors in Toll-like receptor signalling. Nat Rev Immunol. 2007;7(5):353–64.
9. Davis BK, Wen H, Ting JP. The inflammasome NLRs in immunity, inflammation, and associated diseases. Annu Rev Immunol. 2011;29:707–35.

10. Quintin J, Cheng SC, van der Meer JW, Netea MG. Innate immune memory: towards a better understanding of host defense mechanisms. Curr Opin Immunol. 2014;29:1–7.
11. West MA, Heagy W. Endotoxin tolerance: a review. Crit Care Med. 2002;30(1 Supp):S64–73.
12. Schmidt EP, Lee WL, Zemans RL, Yamashita C, Downey GP. On, around, and through: neutrophil-endothelial interactions in innate immunity. Physiol (Bethesda). 2011;26(5):334–47.
13. Studies N-NWGoRiA, Chanock SJ, Manolio T, Boehnke M, Boerwinkle E, Hunter DJ, et al. Replicating genotype-phenotype associations. Nature. 2007;447(7145):655–60.
14. van't Veer LJ, Bernards R. Enabling personalized cancer medicine through analysis of gene-expression patterns. Nature. 2008;452(7187):564–70.
15. Rakyan VK, Down TA, Balding DJ, Beck S. Epigenome-wide association studies for common human diseases. Nat Rev Genet. 2011;12(8):529–41.
16. Michels KB, Binder AM, Dedeurwaerder S, Epstein CB, Greally JM, Gut I, et al. Recommendations for the design and analysis of epigenome-wide association studies. Nat Methods. 2013;10(10):949–55.
17. Sham PC, Purcell SM. Statistical power and significance testing in large-scale genetic studies. Nat Rev Genet. 2014;15(5):335–46.
18. Sims D, Sudbery I, Ilott NE, Heger A, Ponting CP. Sequencing depth and coverage: key considerations in genomic analyses. Nat Rev Genet. 2014;15(2):121–32.
19. Benjamini Y, Hochberg Y. Controlling the false discovery rate: a practical and powerful approach to multiple testing. J R Stat Soc Series B (Methodological). 1995;57(1):289–300.
20. Gerstein M. Genomics: ENCODE leads the way on big data. Nature. 2012;489(7415):208.
21. Harrow J, Frankish A, Gonzalez JM, Tapanari E, Diekhans M, Kokocinski F, et al. GENCODE: the reference human genome annotation for The ENCODE Project. Genome Res. 2012;22(9):1760–74.
22. Roadmap Epigenomics C, Kundaje A, Meuleman W, Ernst J, Bilenky M, Yen A, et al. Integrative analysis of 111 reference human epigenomes. Nature. 2015;518(7539):317–30.
23. Kruglyak L. The road to genome-wide association studies. Nat Rev Genet. 2008;9(4):314–8.
24. Slatkin M. Linkage disequilibrium–understanding the evolutionary past and mapping the medical future. Nat Rev Genet. 2008;9(6):477–85.
25. Welter D, MacArthur J, Morales J, Burdett T, Hall P, Junkins H, et al. The NHGRI GWAS Catalog, a curated resource of SNP-trait associations. Nucleic acids Res. 2014;42(Database issue):D1001–6.
26. Bush WS, Moore JH. Chapter 11: Genome-wide association studies. PLoS Comput Biol. 2012;8(12):e1002822.
27. Altshuler DM, Gibbs RA, Peltonen L, Dermitzakis E, Schaffner SF, Yu F, et al. Integrating common and rare genetic variation in diverse human populations. Nature. 2010;467 (7311):52–8.
28. Abecasis GR, Auton A, Brooks LD, DePristo MA, Durbin RM, Handsaker RE, et al. An integrated map of genetic variation from 1,092 human genomes. Nature. 2012;491 (7422):56–65.
29. Zeggini E, Ioannidis JP. Meta-analysis in genome-wide association studies. Pharmacogenomics. 2009;10(2):191–201.
30. Willer CJ, Li Y, Abecasis GR. METAL: fast and efficient meta-analysis of genomewide association scans. Bioinformatics. 2010;26(17):2190–1.
31. Winkler TW, Day FR, Croteau-Chonka DC, Wood AR, Locke AE, Magi R, et al. Quality control and conduct of genome-wide association meta-analyses. Nat Protoc. 2014;9 (5):1192–212.
32. Howie BN, Donnelly P, Marchini J. A flexible and accurate genotype imputation method for the next generation of genome-wide association studies. PLoS Genet. 2009;5(6):e1000529.
33. Scott LJ, Mohlke KL, Bonnycastle LL, Willer CJ, Li Y, Duren WL, et al. A genome-wide association study of type 2 diabetes in Finns detects multiple susceptibility variants. Science. 2007;316(5829):1341–5.

34. Gibson G. Rare and common variants: twenty arguments. Nat Rev Genet. 2011;13(2):135–45.
35. Cirulli ET, Goldstein DB. Uncovering the roles of rare variants in common disease through whole-genome sequencing. Nat Rev Genet. 2010;11(6):415–25.
36. Wang Q, Lu Q, Zhao H. A review of study designs and statistical methods for genomic epidemiology studies using next generation sequencing. Front Genet. 2015;6:149.
37. Zuk O, Schaffner SF, Samocha K, Do R, Hechter E, Kathiresan S, et al. Searching for missing heritability: designing rare variant association studies. Proc Natl Acad Sci USA. 2014;111(4):E455–64.
38. Lander ES, Linton LM, Birren B, Nusbaum C, Zody MC, Baldwin J, et al. Initial sequencing and analysis of the human genome. Nature. 2001;409(6822):860–921.
39. Venter JC, Adams MD, Myers EW, Li PW, Mural RJ, Sutton GG, et al. The sequence of the human genome. Science. 2001;291(5507):1304–51.
40. Hutchison CA 3rd. DNA sequencing: bench to bedside and beyond. Nucleic Acids Res. 2007;35(18):6227–37.
41. Metzker ML. Sequencing technologies—the next generation. Nat Rev Genet. 2010;11(1):31–46.
42. Thompson JF, Milos PM. The properties and applications of single-molecule DNA sequencing. Genome Biol. 2011;12(2):217.
43. Mamanova L, Coffey AJ, Scott CE, Kozarewa I, Turner EH, Kumar A, et al. Target-enrichment strategies for next-generation sequencing. Nat Methods. 2010;7(2):111–8.
44. Berger B, Peng J, Singh M. Computational solutions for omics data. Nat Rev Genet. 2013;14(5):333–46.
45. Goldstein DB, Allen A, Keebler J, Margulies EH, Petrou S, Petrovski S, et al. Sequencing studies in human genetics: design and interpretation. Nat Rev Genet. 2013;14(7):460–70.
46. Koboldt DC, Ding L, Mardis ER, Wilson RK. Challenges of sequencing human genomes. Brief Bioinform. 11(5):484–98.
47. Nielsen R, Paul JS, Albrechtsen A, Song YS. Genotype and SNP calling from next-generation sequencing data. Nat Rev Genet. 2011;12(6):443–51.
48. McKenna A, Hanna M, Banks E, Sivachenko A, Cibulskis K, Kernytsky A, et al. The genome analysis toolkit: a MapReduce framework for analyzing next-generation DNA sequencing data. Genome Res. 2010;20(9):1297–303.
49. Li H, Handsaker B, Wysoker A, Fennell T, Ruan J, Homer N, et al. The sequence alignment/map format and SAMtools. Bioinformatics. 2009;25(16):2078–9.
50. Lee S, Wu MC, Lin X. Optimal tests for rare variant effects in sequencing association studies. Biostatistics. 2012;13(4):762–75.
51. Kumar P, Henikoff S, Ng PC. Predicting the effects of coding non-synonymous variants on protein function using the SIFT algorithm. Nat Protoc. 2009;4(7):1073–81.
52. Adzhubei IA, Schmidt S, Peshkin L, Ramensky VE, Gerasimova A, Bork P, et al. A method and server for predicting damaging missense mutations. Nat Methods. 2010;7(4):248–9.
53. Wang K, Li M, Hakonarson H. ANNOVAR: functional annotation of genetic variants from high-throughput sequencing data. Nucleic Acids Res. 2010;38(16):e164.
54. Cooper GM, Shendure J. Needles in stacks of needles: finding disease-causal variants in a wealth of genomic data. Nat Rev Genet. 2011;12(9):628–40.
55. Cooper GM, Stone EA, Asimenos G, Green ED, Batzoglou S, Sidow A. Distribution and intensity of constraint in mammalian genomic sequence. Genome Res. 2005;15(7):901–13.
56. Kircher M, Witten DM, Jain P, O'Roak BJ, Cooper GM, Shendure J. A general framework for estimating the relative pathogenicity of human genetic variants. Nat Genet. 2014;46(3):310–5.
57. Kiezun A, Garimella K, Do R, Stitziel NO, Neale BM, McLaren PJ, et al. Exome sequencing and the genetic basis of complex traits. Nat Genet. 2012;44(6):623–30.
58. Cook DN, Pisetsky DS, Schwartz DA. Toll-like receptors in the pathogenesis of human disease. Nat Immunol. 2004;5(10):975–9.

59. Wurfel MM, Gordon AC, Holden TD, Radella F, Strout J, Kajikawa O, et al. Toll-like receptor 1 polymorphisms affect innate immune responses and outcomes in sepsis. Am J Respir Crit Care Med. 2008;178(7):710–20.
60. Mikacenic C, Reiner AP, Holden TD, Nickerson DA, Wurfel MM. Variation in the TLR10/TLR1/TLR6 locus is the major genetic determinant of interindividual difference in TLR1/2-mediated responses. Genes Immun. 2013;14(1):52–7.
61. Reddy AJ, Kleeberger SR. Genetic polymorphisms associated with acute lung injury. Pharmacogenomics. 2009;10(9):1527–39.
62. Shortt K, Chaudhary S, Grigoryev D, Heruth DP, Venkitachalam L, Zhang LQ, et al. Identification of novel single nucleotide polymorphisms associated with acute respiratory distress syndrome by exome-seq. PLoS ONE. 2014;9(11):e111953.
63. Meyer NJ, Li M, Feng R, Bradfield J, Gallop R, Bellamy S, et al. ANGPT2 genetic variant is associated with trauma-associated acute lung injury and altered plasma angiopoietin-2 isoform ratio. Am J Respir Crit Care Med. 2011;183(10):1344–53.
64. Meyer NJ, Feng R, Li M, Zhao Y, Sheu CC, Tejera P, et al. IL1RN coding variant is associated with lower risk of acute respiratory distress syndrome and increased plasma IL-1 receptor antagonist. Am J Respir Crit Care Med. 2013;187(9):950–9.
65. Ahasic AM, Zhao Y, Su L, Sheu CC, Thompson BT, Christiani DC. Adiponectin gene polymorphisms and acute respiratory distress syndrome susceptibility and mortality. PLoS ONE. 2014;9(2):e89170.
66. Brown SM, Grissom CK, Rondina MT, Hoidal JR, Scholand MB, Wolff RK, et al. Polymorphisms in key pulmonary inflammatory pathways and the development of acute respiratory distress syndrome. Exp Lung Res. 2015;41(3):155–62.
67. Wei Y, Wang Z, Su L, Chen F, Tejera P, Bajwa EK, et al. Platelet count mediates the contribution of a genetic variant in LRRC16A to ARDS risk. Chest. 2015;147(3):607–17.
68. Tejera P, Meyer NJ, Chen F, Feng R, Zhao Y, O'Mahony DS, et al. Distinct and replicable genetic risk factors for acute respiratory distress syndrome of pulmonary or extrapulmonary origin. J Med Genet. 2012;49(11):671–80.
69. Johnsson P, Morris KV, Grander D. Pseudogenes: a novel source of trans-acting antisense RNAs. Methods Mol Biol. 2014;1167:213–26.
70. Tay Y, Rinn J, Pandolfi PP. The multilayered complexity of ceRNA crosstalk and competition. Nature. 2014;505(7483):344–52.
71. Esteller M. Non-coding RNAs in human disease. Nat Rev Genet. 2011;12(12):861–74.
72. Leek JT, Scharpf RB, Bravo HC, Simcha D, Langmead B, Johnson WE, et al. Tackling the widespread and critical impact of batch effects in high-throughput data. Nat Rev Genet. 2010;11(10):733–9.
73. Quackenbush J. Computational analysis of microarray data. Nat Rev Genet. 2001;2(6):418–27.
74. Relogio A, Schwager C, Richter A, Ansorge W, Valcarcel J. Optimization of oligonucleotide-based DNA microarrays. Nucleic Acids Res. 2002;30(11):e51.
75. Yang YH, Speed T. Design issues for cDNA microarray experiments. Nat Rev Genet. 2002;3(8):579–88.
76. Allison DB, Cui X, Page GP, Sabripour M. Microarray data analysis: from disarray to consolidation and consensus. Nat Rev Genet. 2006;7(1):55–65.
77. Expression profiling-best practices for data generation and interpretation in clinical trials. Nat Rev Genet. 2004;5(3):229–37.
78. Wang Z, Gerstein M, Snyder M. RNA-Seq: a revolutionary tool for transcriptomics. Nat Rev Genet. 2009;10(1):57–63.
79. Westermann AJ, Gorski SA, Vogel J. Dual RNA-seq of pathogen and host. Nat Rev Microbiol. 2012;10(9):618–30.
80. Treutlein B, Brownfield DG, Wu AR, Neff NF, Mantalas GL, Espinoza FH, et al. Reconstructing lineage hierarchies of the distal lung epithelium using single-cell RNA-seq. Nature. 2014;509(7500):371–5.

81. Kim D, Pertea G, Trapnell C, Pimentel H, Kelley R, Salzberg SL. TopHat2: accurate alignment of transcriptomes in the presence of insertions, deletions and gene fusions. Genome Biol. 2013;14(4):R36.
82. Quinlan AR, Hall IM. BEDTools: a flexible suite of utilities for comparing genomic features. Bioinformatics. 2010;26(6):841–2.
83. Martin JA, Wang Z. Next-generation transcriptome assembly. Nat Rev Genet. 2011;12 (10):671–82.
84. Garber M, Grabherr MG, Guttman M, Trapnell C. Computational methods for transcriptome annotation and quantification using RNA-seq. Nat Methods. 2011;8(6):469–77.
85. Parrish RS, Spencer HJ 3rd. Effect of normalization on significance testing for oligonucleotide microarrays. J Biopharm Stat. 2004;14(3):575–89.
86. Hansen KD, Irizarry RA, Wu Z. Removing technical variability in RNA-seq data using conditional quantile normalization. Biostatistics. 2012;13(2):204–16.
87. Leek JT, Johnson WE, Parker HS, Jaffe AE, Storey JD. The sva package for removing batch effects and other unwanted variation in high-throughput experiments. Bioinformatics. 2012;28(6):882–3.
88. Stegle O, Parts L, Piipari M, Winn J, Durbin R. Using probabilistic estimation of expression residuals (PEER) to obtain increased power and interpretability of gene expression analyses. Nat Protoc. 2012;7(3):500–7.
89. Hunter L, Taylor RC, Leach SM, Simon R. GEST: a gene expression search tool based on a novel Bayesian similarity metric. Bioinformatics. 2001;17(Suppl 1):S115–22.
90. Smyth GK. Linear models and empirical bayes methods for assessing differential expression in microarray experiments. Statistical applications in genetics and molecular biology. 2004;3:Article3.
91. Anders S, Huber W. Differential expression analysis for sequence count data. Genome Biol. 2010;11(10):R106.
92. Robinson MD, McCarthy DJ, Smyth GK. edgeR: a Bioconductor package for differential expression analysis of digital gene expression data. Bioinformatics. 2010;26(1):139–40.
93. Auer PL, Srivastava S, Doerge RW. Differential expression—the next generation and beyond. Briefings Funct Genomics. 2012;11(1):57–62.
94. Trapnell C, Roberts A, Goff L, Pertea G, Kim D, Kelley DR, et al. Differential gene and transcript expression analysis of RNA-seq experiments with TopHat and Cufflinks. Nat Protoc. 2012;7(3):562–78.
95. Stegle O, Teichmann SA, Marioni JC. Computational and analytical challenges in single-cell transcriptomics. Nat Rev Genet. 2015;16(3):133–45.
96. Schmittgen TD, Livak KJ. Analyzing real-time PCR data by the comparative C(T) method. Nat Protoc. 2008;3(6):1101–8.
97. Wurfel MM, Park WY, Radella F, Ruzinski J, Sandstrom A, Strout J, et al. Identification of high and low responders to lipopolysaccharide in normal subjects: an unbiased approach to identify modulators of innate immunity. J Immunol. 2005;175(4):2570–8.
98. Xiao C, Rajewsky K. MicroRNA control in the immune system: basic principles. Cell. 2009;136(1):26–36.
99. Fitzgerald KA, Caffrey DR. Long noncoding RNAs in innate and adaptive immunity. Curr Opin Immunol. 2014;26:140–6.
100. Dolinay T, Kim YS, Howrylak J, Hunninghake GM, An CH, Fredenburgh L, et al. Inflammasome-regulated cytokines are critical mediators of acute lung injury. Am J Respir Crit Care Med. 2012;185(11):1225–34.
101. Kangelaris KN, Prakash A, Liu KD, Aouizerat B, Woodruff PG, Erle DJ, et al. Increased expression of neutrophil-related genes in patients with early sepsis-induced ARDS. Am J Physiol Lung Cell Mol Physiol. 2015:ajplung 00380 2014.
102. Kovach MA, Stringer KA, Bunting R, Wu X, San Mateo L, Newstead MW, et al. Microarray analysis identifies IL-1 receptor type 2 as a novel candidate biomarker in patients with acute respiratory distress syndrome. Respir Res. 2015;16(1):29.

103. Ware LB, Koyama T, Zhao Z, Janz DR, Wickersham N, Bernard GR, et al. Biomarkers of lung epithelial injury and inflammation distinguish severe sepsis patients with acute respiratory distress syndrome. Crit Care. 2013;17(5):R253.

104. Meyer NJ. Beyond single-nucleotide polymorphisms: genetics, genomics, and other 'omic approaches to acute respiratory distress syndrome. Clin Chest Med. 2014;35(4):673–84.

105. Ahmad N, Gerhard GS, Broach JR, Choi AMK, Howrylak JA. Using RNA-seq profiling to identify biomarkers for the acute respiratory distress syndrome (ARDS). Am J Respir Crit Care Med. 2015;191:A1611.

106. Zhou T, Garcia JG, Zhang W. Integrating microRNAs into a system biology approach to acute lung injury. Trans Res: J Lab Clin Med. 2011;157(4):180–90.

107. Dunham I, Kundaje A, Aldred SF, Collins PJ, Davis CA, Doyle F, et al. An integrated encyclopedia of DNA elements in the human genome. Nature. 2012;489(7414):57–74.

108. Allis CD, Jenuwein T, Reinberg D, (Eds). Epigenetics: Cold Spring Harbor Laboratory Press; 2009.

109. Feinberg AP. Phenotypic plasticity and the epigenetics of human disease. Nature. 2007;447 (7143):433–40.

110. Feinberg AP, Tycko B. The history of cancer epigenetics. Nat Rev Cancer. 2004;4(2):143–53.

111. Doi A, Park IH, Wen B, Murakami P, Aryee MJ, Irizarry R, et al. Differential methylation of tissue- and cancer-specific CpG island shores distinguishes human induced pluripotent stem cells, embryonic stem cells and fibroblasts. Nat Gen. 2009;41(12):1350–3.

112. Ji H, Ehrlich LI, Seita J, Murakami P, Doi A, Lindau P, et al. Comprehensive methylome map of lineage commitment from haematopoietic progenitors. Nature. 2010.

113. Jones PA. Functions of DNA methylation: islands, start sites, gene bodies and beyond. Nat Rev Genet. 2012;13(7):484–92.

114. Kulis M, Heath S, Bibikova M, Queiros AC, Navarro A, Clot G, et al. Epigenomic analysis detects widespread gene-body DNA hypomethylation in chronic lymphocytic leukemia. Nat Genet. 2012;44(11):1236–42.

115. Lister R, Pelizzola M, Dowen RH, Hawkins RD, Hon G, Tonti-Filippini J, et al. Human DNA methylomes at base resolution show widespread epigenomic differences. Nature. 2009;462(7271):315–22.

116. Branco MR, Ficz G, Reik W. Uncovering the role of 5-hydroxymethylcytosine in the epigenome. Nat Rev Genet. 2012;13(1):7–13.

117. Schones DE, Zhao K. Genome-wide approaches to studying chromatin modifications. Nat Rev Genet. 2008;9(3):179–91.

118. Ivanov M, Kals M, Kacevska M, Metspalu A, Ingelman-Sundberg M, Milani L. In-solution hybrid capture of bisulfite-converted DNA for targeted bisulfite sequencing of 174 ADME genes. Nucleic Acids Res. 2013;41(6):e72.

119. Li Q, Suzuki M, Wendt J, Patterson N, Eichten SR, Hermanson PJ, et al. Post-conversion targeted capture of modified cytosines in mammalian and plant genomes. Nucleic Acids Res. 2015.

120. Smallwood SA, Lee HJ, Angermueller C, Krueger F, Saadeh H, Peat J, et al. Single-cell genome-wide bisulfite sequencing for assessing epigenetic heterogeneity. Nat Methods. 2014;11(8):817–20.

121. Nazor KL, Boland MJ, Bibikova M, Klotzle B, Yu M, Glenn-Pratola VL, et al. Application of a low cost array-based technique—TAB-Array—for quantifying and mapping both 5mC and 5hmC at single base resolution in human pluripotent stem cells. Genomics. 2014;104 (5):358–67.

122. Yu M, Hon GC, Szulwach KE, Song CX, Zhang L, Kim A, et al. Base-resolution analysis of 5-hydroxymethylcytosine in the mammalian genome. Cell. 2012;149(6):1368–80.

123. Booth MJ, Branco MR, Ficz G, Oxley D, Krueger F, Reik W, et al. Quantitative sequencing of 5-methylcytosine and 5-hydroxymethylcytosine at single-base resolution. Science. 2012;336(6083):934–7.

124. Maksimovic J, Gordon L, Oshlack A. SWAN: Subset-quantile Within Array Normalization for Illumina Infinium HumanMethylation450 BeadChips. Genome Biol. 2012;13(6):R44.

125. Pedersen BS, Schwartz DA, Yang IV, Kechris KJ. Comb-p: software for combining, analyzing, grouping and correcting spatially correlated P-values. Bioinformatics. 2012;28 (22):2986–8.

126. Jaffe AE, Murakami P, Lee H, Leek JT, Fallin MD, Feinberg AP, et al. Bump hunting to identify differentially methylated regions in epigenetic epidemiology studies. Int J Epidemiol. 2012;41(1):200–9.

127. Price ME, Cotton AM, Lam LL, Farre P, Emberly E, Brown CJ, et al. Additional annotation enhances potential for biologically-relevant analysis of the Illumina Infinium HumanMethylation450 BeadChip array. Epigenetics Chromatin. 2013;6(1):4.

128. Houseman EA, Accomando WP, Koestler DC, Christensen BC, Marsit CJ, Nelson HH, et al. DNA methylation arrays as surrogate measures of cell mixture distribution. BMC Bioinform. 2012;13:86.

129. Houseman EA, Molitor J, Marsit CJ. Reference-free cell mixture adjustments in analysis of DNA methylation data. Bioinformatics. 2014;30(10):1431–9.

130. Dupont JM, Tost J, Jammes H, Gut IG. De novo quantitative bisulfite sequencing using the pyrosequencing technology. Anal Biochem. 2004;333(1):119–27.

131. Coolen MW, Statham AL, Gardiner-Garden M, Clark SJ. Genomic profiling of CpG methylation and allelic specificity using quantitative high-throughput mass spectrometry: critical evaluation and improvements. Nucleic Acids Res. 2007;35(18):e119.

132. Roessler J, Ammerpohl O, Gutwein J, Hasemeier B, Anwar SL, Kreipe H, et al. Quantitative cross-validation and content analysis of the 450 k DNA methylation array from Illumina. Inc. BMC Res Notes. 2012;5:210.

133. Arrowsmith CH, Bountra C, Fish PV, Lee K, Schapira M. Epigenetic protein families: a new frontier for drug discovery. Nat Rev Drug Discovery. 2012;11(5):384–400.

134. Tarakhovsky A. Tools and landscapes of epigenetics. Nat Immunol. 2010;11(7):565–8.

135. Rivera CM, Ren B. Mapping human epigenomes. Cell. 2013;155(1):39–55.

136. Kidder BL, Hu G, Zhao K. ChIP-Seq: technical considerations for obtaining high-quality data. Nat Immunol. 2011;12(10):918–22.

137. Landt SG, Marinov GK, Kundaje A, Kheradpour P, Pauli F, Batzoglou S, et al. ChIP-seq guidelines and practices of the ENCODE and modENCODE consortia. Genome Res. 2012;22(9):1813–31.

138. Adli M, Bernstein BE. Whole-genome chromatin profiling from limited numbers of cells using nano-ChIP-seq. Nat Protoc. 2011;6(10):1656–68.

139. Brind'Amour J, Liu S, Hudson M, Chen C, Karimi MM, Lorincz MC. An ultra-low-input native ChIP-seq protocol for genome-wide profiling of rare cell populations. Nature Commun. 2015;6:6033.

140. Furey TS. ChIP-seq and beyond: new and improved methodologies to detect and characterize protein-DNA interactions. Nat Rev Genet. 2012;13(12):840–52.

141. Zhang Y, Liu T, Meyer CA, Eeckhoute J, Johnson DS, Bernstein BE, et al. Model-based analysis of ChIP-Seq (MACS). Genome Biol. 2008;9(9):R137.

142. Mehta S, Jeffrey KL. Beyond receptors and signaling: epigenetic factors in the regulation of innate immunity. Immunol Cell Biol. 2015;93(3):233–44.

143. Stender JD, Glass CK. Epigenomic control of the innate immune response. Curr Opin Pharmacol. 2013;13(4):582–7.

144. Alvarez-Errico D, Vento-Tormo R, Sieweke M, Ballestar E. Epigenetic control of myeloid cell differentiation, identity and function. Nat Rev Immunol. 2015;15(1):7–17.

145. Foster SL, Hargreaves DC, Medzhitov R. Gene-specific control of inflammation by TLR-induced chromatin modifications. Nature. 2007;447(7147):972–8.

146. Saeed S, Quintin J, Kerstens HH, Rao NA, Aghajanirefah A, Matarese F, et al. Epigenetic programming of monocyte-to-macrophage differentiation and trained innate immunity. Science. 2014;345(6204):1251086.
147. Cheng SC, Quintin J, Cramer RA, Shepardson KM, Saeed S, Kumar V, et al. mTOR- and HIF-1alpha-mediated aerobic glycolysis as metabolic basis for trained immunity. Science. 2014;345(6204):1250684.
148. Hawkins RD, Hon GC, Ren B. Next-generation genomics: an integrative approach. Nat Rev Genet. 2010;11(7):476–86.
149. Majewski J, Pastinen T. The study of eQTL variations by RNA-seq: from SNPs to phenotypes. Trends in genetics: TIG. 2011;27(2):72–9.
150. Montgomery SB, Dermitzakis ET. From expression QTLs to personalized transcriptomics. Nat Rev Genet. 2011;12(4):277–82.
151. Ramanan VK, Shen L, Moore JH, Saykin AJ. Pathway analysis of genomic data: concepts, methods, and prospects for future development. Trends Gen TIG. 2012;28(7):323–32.
152. Kramer A, Green J, Pollard J Jr, Tugendreich S. Causal analysis approaches in ingenuity pathway analysis. Bioinformatics. 2014;30(4):523–30.
153. Tarca AL, Draghici S, Khatri P, Hassan SS, Mittal P, Kim JS, et al. A novel signaling pathway impact analysis. Bioinformatics. 2009;25(1):75–82.
154. Langfelder P, Horvath S. WGCNA: an R package for weighted correlation network analysis. BMC Bioinf. 2008;9:559.
155. Subramanian A, Tamayo P, Mootha VK, Mukherjee S, Ebert BL, Gillette MA, et al. Gene set enrichment analysis: a knowledge-based approach for interpreting genome-wide expression profiles. Proc Natl Acad Sci USA. 2005;102(43):15545–50.

Chapter 10
MicroRNA Analysis in Acute Lung Injury

Andrew J. Goodwin

Introduction to MicroRNA

Background

Acute lung injury (ALI), or its clinically defined correlate entity the acute respiratory distress syndrome (ARDS), is an acute inflammatory response in the lungs to either a local (i.e., pneumonia) or systemic (i.e., trauma) insult that may be either infectious or non-infectious. Although ARDS is defined by specific clinical criteria [1] and characterized by a pathologic constellation including epithelial and endothelial injury, proteinaceous alveolar edema, and leukocyte infiltration [2], there is still much unknown about its pathogenesis. This point is well illustrated by epidemiologic data which suggest that less than 10 % of patients who are admitted to the intensive care unit at risk for ARDS go on to develop the condition [3]. Additionally, the clinical course of ALI is highly variable with some patients experiencing a mild course, while others may develop severe injury resulting in death or long-term physical, cognitive, and emotional disability [4, 5]. As such, investigators have exerted considerable effort toward better identification of risk factors for ALI [3] as well as a deeper understanding of its cellular and molecular underpinnings [6].

In the last 10 years, genetic analyses have identified more than 30 DNA polymorphisms that are associated either with ARDS development or outcome [7].

A.J. Goodwin (✉)
Division of Pulmonary, Critical Care, Allergy and Sleep Medicine, Medical University of South Carolina, Suite 816 Clinical Sciences Building, MSC 630, 96 Jonathan Lucas Street, Charleston, SC 29425, USA
e-mail: goodwian@musc.edu

© Springer International Publishing AG 2017
L.M. Schnapp and C. Feghali-Bostwick (eds.), *Acute Lung Injury and Repair*,
Respiratory Medicine, DOI 10.1007/978-3-319-46527-2_10

Many have been validated in more than one population [8–13] and several such as ANGPT2 (angiopoietin 2) [8, 10], SFTPB (surfactant protein B) [11], and IL-10 [9] have strong biological plausibility due to their impact on endothelial, epithelial, and immune cell function. These studies have shed critically important light on potential mechanisms of ALI development and may open the door to the development of novel therapeutic approaches. However, a limitation to genetic association studies using genomic DNA is the inability to analyze epigenetic phenomena which impact gene expression posttranscriptionally. Posttranscriptional gene modification could play key roles in complex, heterogeneous diseases such as ALI and, thus may be an important area of investigation. Here we will focus on the study of one mechanism of post-translational gene modification with considerable promise to shed light on complex disease: micro RNA (miRNA).

MiRNA are 19–25 nucleotide (nt) long segments of non-coding RNA which are known to bind to and inhibit the translation of target mRNA. Over 1800 human miRNA have been identified to date and data suggest that each miRNA has the potential to bind to hundreds of different mRNA targets [14, 15]. Indeed, one study estimates that as much as 60 % of mammalian mRNA are conserved targets for miRNA [16]. As such, miRNA represent a widespread and potentially critical mechanism by which gene expression is regulated. The ability to quantify miRNA expression in cells, tissues and biofluids allows researchers to assess for patterns in diseases of interest and subsequently identify gene targets of potential relevance to the disease. Further, miRNA expression patterns also have the potential to identify those at risk for developing ALI at an early stage before protein expression levels are altered and, therefore, have the capability to serve as either diagnostic or prognostic biomarkers. The remainder of this chapter will provide further background into miRNA and their function as well as discuss various approaches to the study of miRNA in ALI and will summarize the current existing knowledge of miRNA expression in ALI.

MiRNA Synthesis and Processing

The initial description of miRNA occurred in 1993 when Lee et al. identified the small RNA, *lin-4*, which was expressed during *C. elegans* development and was shown to repress protein translation by binding to target mRNA [17]. Subsequently, *let-7* was also identified in *C. elegans* and found to exhibit similar functions [18]. Then in landmark, contemporary studies published in 2001, independent teams of investigators discovered the existence of a much larger pool of miRNA that appeared to be conserved across a wide range of species including humans [19, 20]. Since then, considerable effort has been devoted to understanding not only the roles that miRNA play in human health and disease but also the mechanisms by which miRNA are generated.

From their earliest descriptions, miRNA were frequently identified in the presence of longer ~70 nt RNA strands [17, 18, 21, 22]. This observation combined with the in silico prediction that these longer RNA strands form stem-loop structures [19, 20] led many to believe that miRNA were likely to be derived from these longer precursors in a manner similar to small interfering RNA (siRNA). Ultimately, this hypothesis was proven when investigators demonstrated that these 70 nt strands were processed into ~22 nt strands by Dicer and that loss of Dicer function resulted in a simultaneous loss of miRNA and an accumulation of ~70 nt RNA [23, 24]. Thus, these ~70 nt strands have been given the title precursor miRNA or "pre-miRNA".

Several miRNA gene clusters have been identified in which multiple miRNA genes have been mapped to relatively short genetic loci [19, 20]. MiRNA from these clusters often exhibit similar expression patterns suggesting that their transcription is governed by common regulatory mechanisms. Accordingly, investigators hypothesized that miRNA from these clusters may all derive from the same nascent transcript which would subsequently be processed into individual pre-miRNA. This "step-wise processing" theory was ultimately proven correct through a series of experiments by Lee et al. They identified the presence of longer gene transcripts originating from miRNA gene clusters. When these nascent transcripts were incubated with cell extract, the transcripts were degraded into shorter sequences which corresponded in size to pre-miRNA and mature miRNA and were subsequently identified as such. Thus, these nascent transcripts were termed, primary miRNA or "pri-miRNA". Interestingly, the investigators identified the presence of pri-miRNA not only from miRNA gene clusters but also from single miRNA genes suggesting that step-wise processing may be a ubiquitous step in all miRNA synthesis [25]. This group went on to identify the nuclear RNase III Drosha and its binding partner DiGeorge Syndrome Critical Region 8 (DGCR8) as key proteins in the processing of pri-miRNA into pre-miRNA [26, 27].

As insights into the biosynthesis of miRNA emerged, a remaining question was where in the cell each processing step was occurring. Through in vitro exposure of pri-miRNA to fractionated nuclear and cytoplasmic contents, researchers were able to demonstrate that pri-miRNA are processed into pre-miRNA while inside the nucleus whereas pre-miRNA are processed into mature miRNA in the cytoplasm [25]. Thus, pre-miRNA were likely being shuttled out of the nucleus during miRNA synthesis. Ultimately, exportin 5 (Exp5) was identified as a key nuclear export receptor with a high specificity for pre-miRNA in a Ran guanosine triphosphate (RanGTP)-dependent manner [28]. Once the Exp5-pre-miRNA complex shuttles into the RanGTP-deplete cytoplasm, the pre-miRNA dissociates and is available for processing by Dicer. Interestingly, pre-miRNA export efficiency was impaired for variant pre-miRNA which, when processed, lead to incorrect mature miRNA. This suggests that the exportin 5-mediated shuttling step may provide a measure of quality control during miRNA synthesis. A summary of the miRNA biosynthesis pathway is seen in Fig. 10.1.

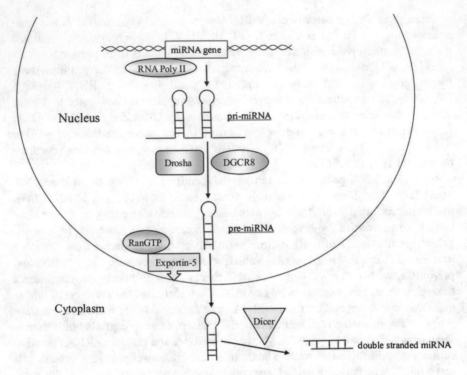

Fig. 10.1 The stepwise biosynthesis of pri-miRNA into double stranded miRNA

MiRNA Function

Upon cleavage of the pre-miRNA by Dicer, the resultant double stranded miRNA associates with the RNA-induced silencing complex (RISC) [29], an incompletely characterized protein complex which includes the RNase argonaute 2 (Ago2) [30]. Once associated, the miRNA duplex is separated into a 5′ strand (guide strand) which is integrated into the RISC [31, 32] and a 3′ strand (passenger strand) [29]. The RISC then uses the guide strand to target mRNA though base pairing with complementary sequences in their 3′ untranslated region (UTR) [33]. Once bound, the mRNA will either: (1) be degraded by Ago2 in the setting of a near perfect match with the miRNA or (2) be prevented from association with ribosomes resulting in inefficient translation in the setting of a partial match with the miRNA [33] (Fig. 10.2). In each case, the net effect is a reduction of protein expression of the targeted gene. It was initially believed that the 3′ strand was degraded by RISC upon separation of the miRNA duplex [29], however, subsequent work has demonstrated that these passenger strands can be functionally active in mRNA targeting as well [34]. Accordingly, miRNA are now designated with a standard nomenclature such that the 5′ strand is given the '5p' suffix while the 3′ strand is given '3p'.

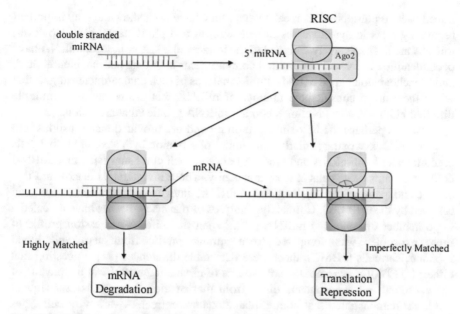

Fig. 10.2 Double stranded miRNA dissociates and couples with the RISC complex resulting in either target mRNA translational repression or complete degradation

The efficiency by which an individual miRNA can recognize and inhibit a target mRNA strand is determined by the complementary match between the miRNA and sequences in the 3′ UTR of the mRNA. Nucleotides 2–7 of the miRNA, known as the miRNA seed, appear to be particularly important as perfect pairing within the seed has been shown to be important for the recognition of most mRNA [34]. Additional pairing outside of the seed including at nucleotide 8 or nucleotides 13–17 of the miRNA have also been shown to increase the efficacy by which it inhibits mRNA translation [35]. Binding site location on the mRNA can also influence a miRNA's ability to repress translation. For instance, binding sites in the 3′ UTR of the mRNA result in more efficient inhibition than do binding sites in translated regions. Further, binding sites that are distant from the center of long UTRs or which are located in regions with concentrated A-U sequences appear to be more susceptible to miRNA targeting [35]. Finally, emerging research has also suggested the existence of miRNA binding sequences within the 5′ UTR of mRNA potentially expanding the number of genes subject to miRNA regulation [36].

Extracellular Compartments Where MiRNA are Located

MiRNA are ubiquitous across cell types and across species of both the plant and animal kingdoms. They have been identified among all cell lineages and can be traced back to pluripotent stem cells where they have been shown to play important regulatory roles in the processes of self-renewal and pluripotency [37]. However, miRNA are not exclusively confined to the intracellular space. Indeed, miRNA have been identified in a variety of biofluid compartments including plasma, pleural fluid, and bronchoalveolar lavage (BAL) fluid. Analyses of each compartment suggest that while there are a considerable number of miRNA that are common to multiple different biofluids, some biofluids contain miRNA profiles that are unique [38].

Plasma is perhaps the best-studied biofluid and has provided many insights into how miRNA exist extracellularly. The initial observation by Valadi et al. that cells could transfer both mRNA and miRNA between each other suggested that miRNA could exist outside of cells at least transiently. These investigators discovered that cells could package RNA, including miRNA, into exosomes which were then released by the cells [39]. Ultimately, analyses of plasma exosomes have revealed a large number of contained miRNA [40]. When the miRNA expression profile of these exosomes was compared to a similar profile from peripheral blood mononuclear cells (PBMC), there were detectable differences [41] suggesting that either: (a) PBMCs were not the sole source of circulating miRNA in the plasma or (b) exosomal miRNA contents differ from that of their donor cells. Subsequent work has demonstrated that both explanations are correct. A variety of cell types have been shown to release exosomal miRNA into the plasma including platelets, endothelial cells, endothelial progenitor cells, and lymphocytes [42–45]. Further, evidence suggests that these cells may release a variety of different vesicles including exosomes, microparticles, microvesicles, and apoptotic bodies [46], each of which may contain miRNA. Additionally, miRNA expression in donor cells and their daughter exosomes often differ [39, 45, 47–49]. The mechanism behind this is incompletely understood and may be related to "selective exportation" of miRNA into the exosomes or differences in the decay kinetics between different miRNA [50, 51].

In addition to vesicle-associated miRNA, investigators have also identified extracellular miRNA which exist outside of membrane-derived particles. This so-called non-vesicle-associated miRNA population appears to be largely protein bound with the RISC component, Ago2, as the predominant extracellular chaperone [52]. When quantified by PCR, this protein bound population appears to account for >90 % of circulating miRNA [52, 53]. Analyses of both the vesicle-associated and non-vesicle-associated miRNA populations have demonstrated that each population is comprised of a distinct pattern of miRNA suggesting that the export systems for each population may differ from each other [54]. Some have suggested that the extracellular protein bound miRNA may derive from the inadvertent release of miRNA during cell death [52], however, this or alternative export mechanisms have not been confirmed.

A third population of extracellular miRNA has been discovered which is bound to circulating high density lipoprotein (HDL) [55]. Similar to theAgo2-bound fraction, the miRNA expression profile in this population was distinct from the vesicle-associated population and has even appeared to differ between disease state and controls. However, the proportion of circulating miRNA which is bound to

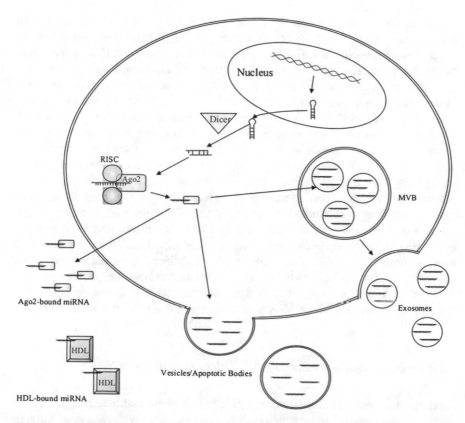

Fig. 10.3 Pre-miRNA are processed into mature miRNA which can remain intracellularly or be exported extracellularly. Extracellular miRNA can be protein bound, HDL-bound, or reside inside of vesicular structures including exosomes and apoptotic bodies. MVB = Multivesicular Body

HDL appears modest raising the question of its functional importance [56]. The different forms of extracellular miRNA are depicted in Fig. 10.3.

Regardless of whether extracellular miRNA are being shuttled inside of exosomes or by proteins, they demonstrate stability both in vivo and in ex vivo storage. Ribonucleases (RNases) in both the bloodstream and the environment commonly degrade large molecular weight RNAs; however, miRNA are typically resistant to this enzymatic cleavage [57]. A portion of this resistance is likely conferred by their association with membrane-derived vesicles or carrier proteins as these may shield the miRNA from enzyme exposure. Indeed, nucleophosmin 1 (NPM1) is a RNA binding protein that has also been implicated as a miRNA shuttle protein and has been shown to protect miRNA from degradation by RNase A [54]. Interestingly, when serum miRNA were exposed to a variety of harsh conditions including boiling, multiple freeze/thaw cycles, low/high pH, and extended storage, they demonstrated remarkable stability suggesting that they may be inherently resistant to degradation as well [57].

Several studies have demonstrated that miRNA can be measured in the alveolar compartment through analysis of BAL fluid [38, 58, 59] and over 200 individual miRNA have been identified in this compartment to date [38]. Unlike some biofluids, BAL does not appear to contain miRNA that are unique only to that compartment but rather it appears to express a subpopulation of miRNA that are found in other compartments including plasma. It is not clear, however, if BAL contains fewer individual miRNA than plasma because certain miRNA are selectively filtered out before entering the alveolar space or because bronchoalveolar cells express and release miRNA in different patterns than circulating or endovascular cells. It is also worth acknowledging that new miRNA are continuously being discovered; thus, miRNA that are unique to the alveolar space with physiologic relevance to pulmonary disease may exist but have yet to be identified. At least two studies have compared expression patterns of miRNA in the BAL between control humans and humans with disease. The first study examined exosomal miRNA expression in both asthmatics and healthy controls and identified a signature of 16 miRNA whose expression levels allowed for classification of the subjects with asthma [58]. The second study reported differential expression patterns of total BAL miRNA between patients with dyspnea and healthy controls and identified correlations between BAL miRNA levels and pulmonary function testing [59].

Cell-to-Cell Communication via Extracellular MiRNA

Since the discovery of extracellular miRNA, investigators have sought to determine whether it is a mechanism by which cells can communicate with each other through manipulation of target cell gene expression. Indeed, numerous examples have now been described in which membrane-derived vesicles containing miRNA have been taken up by recipient cells leading to altered target gene expression and/or cellular function [39, 43, 45, 47, 60–62]. Hergenreider et al. [62] found endothelial cells placed under shear stress released miRNA-filled vesicles which, in turn, were internalized by cocultured vascular smooth muscle cells resulting in alterations in their gene expression. Similarly, Zernecke and colleagues demonstrated that apoptotic endothelial cells can release vesicular apoptotic bodies which contain, among others, miR-126 and are internalized by adjacent endothelial cells. Through a series of elegant experiments using apoptotic bodies from control and miR-126 deficient mice, they showed that delivery of miR-126 induced expression of the chemokine CXCL12 and attenuated the development of atherosclerosis [43].

Non-vesicle-associated miRNA may also serve as a mechanism for cell-to-cell communication. For example, HDL-bound miRNA can be effectively delivered to hepatocytes in vitro with resultant alterations in hepatocyte gene expression [55]. This mode of delivery is dependent upon scavenger receptor class B type I, however, and may not occur in all cell types. Indeed, similar uptake has not been demonstrated in endothelial cells, smooth muscle cells, or PBMCs suggesting that HDL-miRNA complexes play only a limited role in cell-to-cell transport of miRNA [56]. Although they represent the largest fraction of extracellular miRNA, it is unclear at this time if Ago2-bound miRNA can be internalized in a manner similar to HDL-bound miRNA or vesicle-associated miRNA. The *C. Elegans* transmembrane channel, SID-1, facilitates the uptake of double stranded RNA including long hairpin miRNA precursors [63, 64]. However, while mammalian homologs of SID-1 exist [65], it is unclear if they can import precursor or mature miRNA, particularly when bound to a protein. Recent investigations which demonstrate that miRNA can bind to and activate extracellular toll-like receptors (TLR) suggest a potential alternative mechanism by which Ago2-bound miRNA can facilitate cell-to-cell communication [66, 67]. Further investigation into the potential roles of non-canonical actions of extracellular miRNA in cell-to-cell communication is warranted.

MicroRNA Analysis in Acute Lung Injury

Background

The heterogeneous nature of ALI suggests that its etiology is likely complex and multifactorial. This is exemplified by its multitude of risk factors, its variable clinical course and by the wide range of genetic associations that have been identified to date [7]. Accordingly, there is inherent appeal to the investigation of miRNA as both an etiologic factor and as a possible therapeutic in ALI given their ability to target many pathways simultaneously, their ubiquitous nature and their ability to facilitate inter-cell communication. As such, investigators have begun to analyze miRNA expression patterns in experimental ALI in order to better understand their potential role in this disease.

At present there are several commercially available array-based approaches for measuring miRNA in both experimental and human disease (Table 10.1). They can be broadly categorized based on the underlying technology that they utilize which include quantitative PCR, hybridization, and sequencing. These arrays are developed based on existing miRNA sequence libraries, most commonly miRbase [14] and are often available either as whole miRnome arrays or as disease or pathway-specific arrays. Each platform has slightly different sample size requirements and performance characteristics when compared head-to-head [68], thus, choosing the optimal array depends upon the needs of the specific study. Alternatively, candidate miRNA approaches using quantitative PCR are also feasible as primers for most miRNA are commercially available.

Potential Applications

Theoretically, miRNA analyses in ALI could focus on several different aspects of the disease. Acute lung injury represents a complex interplay between the immune

Table 10.1 Commercially available miRNA arrays

Platform	Company	Technology	Species Available	Required RNA amount (ng)
GeneChip miRNA array	Affymetrix	Hybridization	Human, mouse, rat	130
miRNA Microarray	Agilent	Hybridization	Human, mouse, rat	100
miRCURY LNA	Exiqon	Quantitative PCR	Human, mouse, rat	250
TruSeq	Illumina	Sequencing	Human, mouse	1000
Ion Torrent	Life Technologies	Sequencing	Human, mouse, rat	1000
Open Array	Life Technologies	Quantitative PCR	Human, mouse, rat	100
Taqman Cards	Life Technologies	Quantitative PCR	Human, mouse, rat	350
nCounter	Nanostring	Hybridization	Human, mouse, rat	100
miScript	Qiagen	Quantitative PCR	Human, mouse, rat, dog, rhesus	500
qScript	Quanta	Quantitative PCR	Human	800
SmartChip	Wafergen	Quantitative PCR	Human	1000

response to an inflammatory insult, endothelial activation/dysfunction, and epithelial injury; and the etiologies of each of these processes, and their interaction with each other, could be investigated through analysis of miRNA expression. As miRNA are upstream regulators of protein expression, they have the potential to exhibit alterations in expression before resultant alterations in protein expression. Thus, miRNA may represent an attractive class of diagnostic biomarkers with the ability to detect patients at risk for ALI before its development. Additionally, with the advent of commercially available miRNA mimics and blockmirs [69], gain or loss of function studies can be performed to determine the impact of individual miRNA on cell function in ALI. Ultimately, as the role of miRNA in ALI is clarified, sophisticated delivery approaches may be employed in order to develop miRNA-based therapeutics.

Bioinformatics

Although previous work has identified direct target interactions for a number of miRNA, the sheer volume of miRNA that have been discovered combined with the knowledge that each miRNA may have dozens to hundreds of targets necessitates a robust bioinformatics approach to interpreting miRNA expression data. Thus, a key component of miRNA research is in silico prediction of miRNA targets and pathway analysis. Several publically available search engines have been developed which use existing knowledge on miRNA-mRNA interactions in order to predict potential targets for miRNA [70, 71]. Most algorithms begin with an analysis of the seed region of the miRNA and the 3′ UTR of mRNA where those mRNA with high complementarity are given a higher score. Next, the 3′ UTR binding site is assessed for conservation across species as higher degrees of conservation have been shown to reduce false positive interactions [72]. Finally, some algorithms evaluate candidate pairings for thermodynamic stability [73] and/or measure the free energy of binding sites [74] in order to further refine the prediction score. As different algorithms often yield substantial differences in predicted targets [75], a prudent approach is to assess for commonality across multiple different algorithms in order to reduce the rate of false positives.

In addition to target prediction, some available software also provide pathway analysis to better understand a miRNA's potential impact on cellular function and to understand if multiple miRNA may have synergistic or antagonistic effects on cell function. Examples of this software include DIANA-miRPath and Ingenuity Pathway Analysis [76, 77]. DIANA-miRPath allows users to assess for predicted targets in either the Tarbase or DIANA microT-CDS databases and then maps identified targets onto molecular pathways using the Kyoto Encyclopedia of Genes and Genomes (KEGG) database. Multiple miRNA can be analyzed simultaneously in order to determine if miRNA of interest potentially act on the same pathways. Ingenuity Pathway Analysis provides similar functionality and allows for reverse prediction where mRNA of interest can be used to predict which miRNA may target them. Target prediction and pathway analysis are often the initial approaches used to examine the potential relevance of differentially expressed miRNA within a specific disease.

Limitations

Although there are numerous potential advantages to analyzing miRNA in ALI, there are also important limitations to consider. An ideal strategy when interpreting miRNA expression data is to simultaneously measure the expression of its downstream targets at both the mRNA and protein level in order to measure its functional impact. This represents a significant challenge in patients with ALI as they seldom undergo lung biopsy, mRNA is not stable in the circulation or alveolar space, and many proteins of interest may not be secreted extracellularly. Thus, the ability to comprehensively assess the impact of miRNA in human ALI in vivo is often limited to cells that can be easily collected from the intravascular or intra alveolar spaces or to proteins secreted into these spaces. Therefore, there is a heavy reliance upon in vitro studies to investigate the potential impact of miRNA on human endothelial and epithelial cells. While animal models of ALI may be used to examine the role of miRNA in vivo as they allow for access to lung tissue, many miRNA (or their targets) are not conserved across species which may limit the ability to apply the knowledge gained from an animal model to human ALI.

An additional challenge encountered in miRNA research in ALI is identifying the cellular source of identified miRNA. As previously discussed, a wide variety of cells release both vesicle-associated and non-vesicle-associated miRNA into the circulation. Additionally, the expression patterns of miRNA inside of exosomes commonly differ from the expression patterns of the originating cells [39, 45, 47–49] adding an extra layer of complexity. While exosomal membranes share protein markers from their donor cells, many of these are nonspecific and do not clarify the origin of the exosome. Future techniques which can purify exosomes and identify their source will help to significantly improve the current ability to interpret circulating miRNA expression patterns and the contribution that different cells play in the circulating miRnome.

Current Knowledge of MiRNA in ALI

The exploration of miRNA expression and their role in ALI is still in its infancy. The currently available literature has focused largely on the expression of miRNA in lung tissue in experimental models of ALI and has suggested that miRNA may help to regulate inflammation and vascular integrity in the setting of ALI. Specifically, in a high tidal volume murine model of ventilator induced lung injury (VILI), several miRNA including miR-146, miR-155, and miR-21, were differentially expressed in lung tissue when compared to lungs ventilated with low tidal volumes. In silico analysis identified that miR-146 and miR-155 regulate central nodes in both TGF-β signaling and inflammatory cytokine pathways in this model. Further, pretreatment with intratracheal anti-miR-21 resulted in improved oxygenation and respiratory mechanics as well as reduced BAL protein levels in response to high tidal volume ventilation [78]. The potential role of miR-146 in ALI was again suggested in a rat model of LPS-induced ALI which demonstrated that miR-146 was upregulated in both lung tissue and alveolar macrophages in the setting of ALI. The investigators also identified that miR-146 functionally suppressed TNF-α, IL-6, and IL-1β expression in alveolar macrophages through the inhibition of IRAK-1 and TRAF-6, key mediators in toll-like receptor signaling [79]. Additionally, delivery of miR-146a to murine ALI has been shown to promote M2 polarization of alveolar macrophages [80]. This suggests that miR-146 may be overexpressed in ALI in an attempt to regulate macrophage function and inflammatory cytokine expression. In contrast, promotion of the M2 phenotype occurs with inhibition of miR-155 using antisense oligonucleotides. MiR-155 inhibition simultaneously reduced BAL cell and protein levels and enhanced clinical recovery from ALI [81].

MicroRNA-16 may also regulate the inflammatory response of ALI in epithelial cells. Cai et al. discovered that miR-16 is down regulated in murine lung tissue after LPS-induced lung injury. When the investigators delivered a miR-16 mimic to A549 epithelial cells in vitro, they found that IL-6 and TNF-α expression decreased suggesting that miR-16 regulates their expression either directly or indirectly.

Bioinformatic analysis suggested potential binding sites for miR-16 in the 3′ UTR of both IL-6 and TNF-α mRNA and ultimately in vitro studies confirmed a direct interaction between miR-16 and the TNF-α 3′ UTR [82]. Thus, miR-16 down-regulation in ALI may contribute to ALI inflammation by releasing TNF-α inhibition.

In addition to modulating the inflammatory response in ALI, miRNA may also influence endothelial activation and dysfunction in this syndrome. While investigating the beneficial effects of human endothelial progenitor cells (EPCs) and a CXCL12 analogue in murine sepsis, investigators discovered that these two therapies can synergistically improve survival and reduce ALI [44]. Simultaneously, intravenous treatment with EPCs altered the expression of endothelial-relevant circulating miRNA, an effect which was accentuated by synergistic treatment with the CXCL12 analogue. Specifically, miR-126 expression, which has pleiotropic, beneficial effects on endothelial homeostasis [43, 83–85], was augmented by treatment with the chemokine analogue. Additionally, miR-155 and miR-34a, which lead to endothelial apoptosis through targeting of Sirt1, both exhibited decreased expression in the blood. Taken together, these data suggest that EPCs (a) may reduce vascular leak through the delivery of exosomes which facilitate the transfer of beneficial miRNA to injured endothelium and that (b) cotreatment with the CXCL12 analogue may enhance this effect by favorably altering the miRNA expression patterns in exosomes [44, 86]. Recent data demonstrating that mesenchymal stem cells (MSC) also exert beneficial effects in ALI via exosomes [87] support this conceptual framework and suggest that nanoparticle delivery of exosomal contents may have therapeutic potential.

Future Directions

Considerable work remains in the study of miRNA in ALI. Although miRNA expression has been studied in animal models of ALI, little is known about their expression in human ALI. Characterizing miRNA expression in both the circulation and the BAL will be critical steps to understanding the potential role of miRNA in human disease. Accordingly, further refinement in techniques which distinguish the cellular origins of specific exosomes will allow investigators to untangle the complex web of circulating miRNA and how they participate in cell-to-cell communication. As this data emerges, in silico target prediction can be coupled with in vitro experimentation to map out how miRNA influence both injury and repair in ALI.

Perhaps the most exciting work to be done in the investigation of miRNA in ALI will be the development of novel miRNA-based therapeutics. As miRNA have many potential gene targets, they are ideally suited to treat complex disorders which involve multiple molecular pathways. Additionally, their stability inside of exosomes provides the potential to package them inside of synthetic nanoparticles which can be targeted to specific cell types of interest [88]. Alternatively, endogenous miRNA expression can be manipulated through delivery of nanoparticle associated blockmirs [89]. As our understanding of the etiologic role of miRNA in ALI improves, we may one day look forward to nanoparticle-based therapy which can modulate the various derangements in the inflammatory response, endothelial integrity, and epithelial function and survival that characterize this disease.

References

1. Force ADT, et al. Acute respiratory distress syndrome: the Berlin Definition. JAMA. 2012;307(23):2526–33.
2. Ware LB, Matthay MA. The acute respiratory distress syndrome. N Engl J Med. 2000;342 (18):1334–49.
3. Gajic O, et al. Early identification of patients at risk of acute lung injury: evaluation of lung injury prediction score in a multicenter cohort study. Am J Respir Crit Care Med. 2011;183 (4):462–70.
4. Hopkins RO, et al. Two-year cognitive, emotional, and quality-of-life outcomes in acute respiratory distress syndrome. Am J Respir Crit Care Med. 2005;171(4):340–7.
5. Herridge MS, et al. Functional disability 5 years after acute respiratory distress syndrome. N Engl J Med. 2011;364(14):1293–304.
6. Matthay MA, Zimmerman GA. Acute lung injury and the acute respiratory distress syndrome: four decades of inquiry into pathogenesis and rational management. Am J Respir Cell Mol Biol. 2005;33(4):319–27.
7. Meyer NJ. Future clinical applications of genomics for acute respiratory distress syndrome. Lancet Respir Med. 2013;1(10):793–803.
8. Meyer NJ, et al. ANGPT2 genetic variant is associated with trauma-associated acute lung injury and altered plasma angiopoietin-2 isoform ratio. Am J Respir Crit Care Med. 2011;183 (10):1344–53.
9. Gong MN, et al. Interleukin-10 polymorphism in position -1082 and acute respiratory distress syndrome. Eur Respir J. 2006;27(4):674–81.
10. van der Heijden M, et al. Angiopoietin-2, permeability oedema, occurrence and severity of ALI/ARDS in septic and non-septic critically ill patients. Thorax. 2008;63(10):903–9.
11. Currier PF, et al. Surfactant protein-B polymorphisms and mortality in the acute respiratory distress syndrome. Crit Care Med. 2008;36(9):2511–6.
12. Marshall RP, et al. Angiotensin converting enzyme insertion/deletion polymorphism is associated with susceptibility and outcome in acute respiratory distress syndrome. Am J Respir Crit Care Med. 2002;166(5):646–50.
13. Medford AR, et al. Vascular endothelial growth factor gene polymorphism and acute respiratory distress syndrome. Thorax. 2005;60(3):244–8.
14. miRBase: the microRNA database. Available from: http://www.mirbase.org/.
15. Lewis BP, Burge CB, Bartel DP. Conserved seed pairing, often flanked by adenosines, indicates that thousands of human genes are microRNA targets. Cell. 2005;120(1):15–20.
16. Friedman RC, et al. Most mammalian mRNAs are conserved targets of microRNAs. Genome Res. 2009;19(1):92–105.
17. Lee RC, Feinbaum RL, Ambros V. The C. elegans heterochronic gene lin-4 encodes small RNAs with antisense complementarity to lin-14. Cell. 1993;75(5):843–54.
18. Reinhart BJ, et al. The 21-nucleotide let-7 RNA regulates developmental timing in Caenorhabditis elegans. Nature. 2000;403(6772):901–6.

19. Lagos-Quintana M, et al. Identification of novel genes coding for small expressed RNAs. Science. 2001;294(5543):853–8.
20. Lau NC, et al. An abundant class of tiny RNAs with probable regulatory roles in Caenorhabditis elegans. Science. 2001;294(5543):858–62.
21. Pasquinelli AE, et al. Conservation of the sequence and temporal expression of let-7 heterochronic regulatory RNA. Nature. 2000;408(6808):86–9.
22. Grishok A, et al. Genes and mechanisms related to RNA interference regulate expression of the small temporal RNAs that control C. elegans developmental timing. Cell. 2001;106 (1):23–34.
23. Ketting RF, et al. Dicer functions in RNA interference and in synthesis of small RNA involved in developmental timing in C. elegans. Genes Dev. 2001;15(20):2654–9.
24. Knight SW, Bass BL. A role for the RNase III enzyme DCR-1 in RNA interference and germ line development in Caenorhabditis elegans. Science. 2001;293(5538):2269–71.
25. Lee Y, et al. MicroRNA maturation: stepwise processing and subcellular localization. EMBO J. 2002;21(17):4663–70.
26. Lee Y, et al. The nuclear RNase III Drosha initiates microRNA processing. Nature. 2003;425 (6956):415–9.
27. Han J, et al. The Drosha-DGCR8 complex in primary microRNA processing. Genes Dev. 2004;18(24):3016–27.
28. Lund E, et al. Nuclear export of microRNA precursors. Science. 2004;303(5654):95–8.
29. Gregory RI, et al. Human RISC couples microRNA biogenesis and posttranscriptional gene silencing. Cell. 2005;123(4):631–40.
30. Meister G. Argonaute proteins: functional insights and emerging roles. Nat Rev Genet. 2013;14(7):447–59.
31. Siomi H, Siomi MC. On the road to reading the RNA-interference code. Nature. 2009;457 (7228):396–404.
32. Preall JB, et al. Short interfering RNA strand selection is independent of dsRNA processing polarity during RNAi in Drosophila. Curr Biol. 2006;16(5):530–5.
33. Pratt AJ, MacRae IJ. The RNA-induced silencing complex: a versatile gene-silencing machine. J Biol Chem. 2009;284(27):17897–901.
34. Bartel DP. MicroRNAs: target recognition and regulatory functions. Cell. 2009;136(2): 215–33.
35. Grimson A, et al. MicroRNA targeting specificity in mammals: determinants beyond seed pairing. Mol Cell. 2007;27(1):91–105.
36. Lee I, et al. New class of microRNA targets containing simultaneous 5'-UTR and 3'-UTR interaction sites. Genome Res. 2009;19(7):1175–83.
37. Lakshmipathy U, Davila J, Hart RP. miRNA in pluripotent stem cells. Regen Med. 2010;5 (4):545–55.
38. Weber JA, et al. The microRNA spectrum in 12 body fluids. Clin Chem. 2010;56(11): 1733–41.
39. Valadi H, et al. Exosome-mediated transfer of mRNAs and microRNAs is a novel mechanism of genetic exchange between cells. Nat Cell Biol. 2007;9(6):654–9.
40. Exosome protein, RNA and lipid database. Available from: www.exocarta.org.
41. Hunter MP, et al. Detection of microRNA expression in human peripheral blood microvesicles. PLoS ONE. 2008;3(11):e3694.
42. Pan Y, et al. Platelet-secreted microRNA-223 promotes endothelial cell apoptosis induced by advanced glycation end products via targeting the insulin-like growth factor 1 receptor. J Immunol. 2014;192(1):437–46.
43. Zernecke A, et al. Delivery of microRNA-126 by apoptotic bodies induces CXCL12-dependent vascular protection. Sci Signal. 2009;2(100):ra81.
44. Fan H, et al. Endothelial progenitor cells and a stromal cell-derived factor-1α analogue synergistically improve survival in sepsis. Am J Respir Crit Care Med. 2014;189(12): 1509–19.

45. Mittelbrunn M, et al. Unidirectional transfer of microRNA-loaded exosomes from T cells to antigen-presenting cells. Nat Commun. 2011;2:282.
46. Thery C, Ostrowski M, Segura E. Membrane vesicles as conveyors of immune responses. Nat Rev Immunol. 2009;9(8):581–93.
47. Skog J, et al. Glioblastoma microvesicles transport RNA and proteins that promote tumour growth and provide diagnostic biomarkers. Nat Cell Biol. 2008;10(12):1470–6.
48. Collino F, et al. Microvesicles derived from adult human bone marrow and tissue specific mesenchymal stem cells shuttle selected pattern of miRNAs. PLoS ONE. 2010;5(7):e11803.
49. Pigati L, et al. Selective release of microRNA species from normal and malignant mammary epithelial cells. PLoS ONE. 2010;5(10):e13515.
50. Bail S, et al. Differential regulation of microRNA stability. RNA. 2010;16(5):1032–9.
51. Krol J, Loedige I, Filipowicz W. The widespread regulation of microRNA biogenesis, function and decay. Nat Rev Genet. 2010;11(9):597–610.
52. Turchinovich A, et al. Characterization of extracellular circulating microRNA. Nucleic Acids Res. 2011;39(16):7223–33.
53. Arroyo JD, et al. Argonaute2 complexes carry a population of circulating microRNAs independent of vesicles in human plasma. Proc Natl Acad Sci USA. 2011;108(12):5003–8.
54. Wang K, et al. Export of microRNAs and microRNA-protective protein by mammalian cells. Nucleic Acids Res. 2010;38(20):7248–59.
55. Vickers KC, et al. MicroRNAs are transported in plasma and delivered to recipient cells by high-density lipoproteins. Nat Cell Biol. 2011;13(4):423–33.
56. Wagner J, et al. Characterization of levels and cellular transfer of circulating lipoprotein-bound microRNAs. Arterioscler Thromb Vasc Biol. 2013;33(6):1392–400.
57. Chen X, et al. Characterization of microRNAs in serum: a novel class of biomarkers for diagnosis of cancer and other diseases. Cell Res. 2008;18(10):997–1006.
58. Levanen B, et al. Altered microRNA profiles in bronchoalveolar lavage fluid exosomes in asthmatic patients. J Allergy Clin Immunol. 2013;131(3):894–903.
59. Brown JN, et al. Protein and microRNA biomarkers from lavage, urine, and serum in military personnel evaluated for dyspnea. BMC Med Genomics. 2014;7:58.
60. Kosaka N, et al. Secretory mechanisms and intercellular transfer of microRNAs in living cells. J Biol Chem. 2010;285(23):17442–52.
61. Montecalvo A, et al. Mechanism of transfer of functional microRNAs between mouse dendritic cells via exosomes. Blood. 2012;119(3):756–66.
62. Hergenreider E, et al. Atheroprotective communication between endothelial cells and smooth muscle cells through miRNAs. Nat Cell Biol. 2012;14(3):249–56.
63. Feinberg EH, Hunter CP. Transport of dsRNA into cells by the transmembrane protein SID-1. Science. 2003;301(5639):1545–7.
64. Shih JD, Hunter CP. SID-1 is a dsRNA-selective dsRNA-gated channel. RNA. 2011;17(6):1057–65.
65. Duxbury MS, Ashley SW, Whang EE. RNA interference: a mammalian SID-1 homologue enhances siRNA uptake and gene silencing efficacy in human cells. Biochem Biophys Res Commun. 2005;331(2):459–63.
66. Fabbri M, et al. MicroRNAs bind to Toll-like receptors to induce prometastatic inflammatory response. Proc Natl Acad Sci USA. 2012;109(31):E2110–6.
67. Lehmann SM, et al. An unconventional role for miRNA: let-7 activates Toll-like receptor 7 and causes neurodegeneration. Nat Neurosci. 2012;15(6):827–35.
68. Mestdagh P, et al. Evaluation of quantitative miRNA expression platforms in the microRNA quality control (miRQC) study. Nat Methods. 2014;11(8):809–15.
69. Young JA, et al. Regulation of vascular leak and recovery from ischemic injury by general and VE-cadherin-restricted miRNA antagonists of miR-27. Blood. 2013;122(16):2911–9.
70. microRNA.org—Targets and Expression. Available from: http://www.microrna.org/microrna/home.do.
71. TargetScanHuman: Prediction of microRNA targets. Available from: http://www.targetscan.org/.

72. Lewis BP, et al. Prediction of mammalian microRNA targets. Cell. 2003;115(7):787–98.
73. Wuchty S, et al. Complete suboptimal folding of RNA and the stability of secondary structures. Biopolymers. 1999;49(2):145–65.
74. Kiriakidou M, et al. A combined computational-experimental approach predicts human microRNA targets. Genes Dev. 2004;18(10):1165–78.
75. Doench JG, Sharp PA. Specificity of microRNA target selection in translational repression. Genes Dev. 2004;18(5):504–11.
76. DIANA miRPath.
77. Ingenuity Pathway Analysis—microRNA Research.
78. Vaporidi K, et al. Pulmonary microRNA profiling in a mouse model of ventilator-induced lung injury. Am J Physiol Lung Cell Mol Physiol. 2012;303(3):L199–207.
79. Zeng Z, et al. Upregulation of miR-146a contributes to the suppression of inflammatory responses in LPS-induced acute lung injury. Exp Lung Res. 2013;39(7):275–82.
80. Vergadi E, et al. Akt2 deficiency protects from acute lung injury via alternative macrophage activation and miR-146a induction in mice. J Immunol. 2014;192(1):394–406.
81. Guo Z, et al. Antisense oligonucleotide treatment enhances the recovery of acute lung injury through IL-10-secreting M2-like macrophage-induced expansion of CD4+ regulatory T cells. J Immunol. 2013;190(8):4337–48.
82. Cai ZG, et al. MicroRNAs are dynamically regulated and play an important role in LPS-induced lung injury. Can J Physiol Pharmacol. 2012;90(1):37–43.
83. Fish JE, et al. miR-126 regulates angiogenic signaling and vascular integrity. Dev Cell. 2008;15(2):272–84.
84. Wang S, et al. The endothelial-specific microRNA miR-126 governs vascular integrity and angiogenesis. Dev Cell. 2008;15(2):261–71.
85. Harris TA, et al. MicroRNA-126 regulates endothelial expression of vascular cell adhesion molecule 1. Proc Natl Acad Sci USA. 2008;105(5):1516–21.
86. Witzenrath M. Endothelial progenitor cells for acute respiratory distress syndrome treatment: support your local sheriff! Am J Respir Crit Care Med. 2014;189(12):1452–5.
87. Monsel A, et al. Therapeutic Effects of Human Mesenchymal Stem Cell-Derived Microvesicles in Severe Pneumonia in Mice. Am J Respir Crit Care Med. 2015;192:324–36.
88. Chen Y, et al. Nanoparticles modified with tumor-targeting scFv deliver siRNA and miRNA for cancer therapy. Mol Ther. 2010;18(9):1650–6.
89. Babar IA, et al. Nanoparticle-based therapy in an in vivo microRNA-155 (miR-155)-dependent mouse model of lymphoma. Proc Natl Acad Sci USA. 2012;109(26):E1695–704.

Index

Note: Page numbers followed by f and t indicate figures and tables, respectively.

© Springer International Publishing AG 2017
L.M. Schnapp and C. Feghali-Bostwick (eds.), *Acute Lung Injury and Repair*,
Respiratory Medicine, DOI 10.1007/978-3-319-46527-2

Printed in the United States
By Bookmasters